WABASH CARNEGIE P LIB

1230 9100 228 408 6

617.5 Old
Foot & ankle pain : self-
treatment for foot and ankle
pain, heel spurs, plantar
fasciitis, assessing shoe inserts
and other diagnoses
Olderman, Rick.

WITHDRAWN

FIXING YOU®

D1526362

BOOKS IN THE **FIXING YOU**®SERIES:

FIXING YOU:®

FOOT &
ANKLE PAIN

SELF-TREATMENT FOR
FOOT AND ANKLE PAIN,
HEEL SPURS, PLANTAR FASCIITIS,
ASSESSING SHOE INSERTS
AND OTHER DIAGNOSES.

RICK OLDERMAN
MSPT, CPT

BOONE
PUBLISHING, LLC

2012 Boone Publishing, LLC

WABASH CARNEGIE PUBLIC LIBRARY

Boone Publishing, LLC

Editor: Lauren Manoy
Layout & Design: Barbara Patterson
(barbara@barbarapattersondesign.com)
Medical Illustrations: Martin Huber (mdhuber@gmail.com),
Meghan Shoemaker (medical_art@yahoo.com)
Exercise Photographs: MaryLynn Gillaspie Photography
(marylynn@mxvphoto.com)

Copyright 2012 by Boone Publishing, LLC

All rights reserved. No part of this publication may be reproduced or transmitted in any form or by any means, electronic or mechanical, including photocopy, recording, or any information storage and retrieval system, without permission in writing from the publisher.

Boone Publishing, LLC
www.BoonePublishing.com

Library of Congress Control Number: 2011961970

Library of Congress Subject Heading:
1. Foot Pain—Physical Therapy—Treatment—Handbooks, manuals, etc. 2.Foot Pain—Physical Therapy—Treatment—Handbooks, manuals, etc. 3. Foot Pain—Popular Works. 4. Foot Pain—Popular Works 5. Foot —Care & Hygiene—Popular Works. 6. Foot —Care & Hygiene—Popular Works. 7. Foot Pain—Exercise Therapy. 8. Foot Pain—Exercise Therapy. 9. Self-care, Health—Handbooks, manuals, etc. 10. Foot Pain—Alternative Treatment. 11. Foot Pain—Alternative Treatment. 12. Foot Pain—Exercise Therapy. 13. Foot Pain—Exercise Therapy. 14. Foot Pain—Prevention. 15. Foot Pain—Prevention. I. Title: Fixing you: foot & ankle pain. II. Olderman, Rick. III. Title.

ISBN 978-0-9821937-5-4

Printed in the United States of America

Version 1.0

ACKNOWLEDGEMENTS

In science and medicine we build on the shoulders of those who have discovered truths before us. Writing the *Fixing You* series has been no different. I would like to deeply thank Dr. Shirley A. Sahrmann for her breakthrough text: *Diagnosis and Treatment of Movement Impairment Syndromes* on which the subject of this series is based. Were it not for her textbook and seminars, which I have immensely enjoyed, I would not have been able to write the *Fixing You* series much less help so many people with their chronic pain or injuries. Dr. Sahrmann is a rare breed with a sharp mind and wit to match. Her depth of knowledge in all things musculoskeletal or movement related leaves me speechless.

Additionally I would like to thank Florence Kendall, Elizabeth McCreary and Patricia Provance for their classic, *Muscles Testing and Function,* fourth edition. This book has been a tectonic plate on which our understanding of orthopedic physical therapy stands.

Lastly I would like to acknowledge the importance of Thomas Hanna's work in understanding pain patterns in the human body. His book, *Somatics: reawakening the mind's control of movement, flexibility, and health* has been instrumental in broadening my understanding of pain and how to help people fix it.

THANK YOU!

I would like to thank Lauren Manoy for painstakingly editing this book. She has meticulously sifted through this information and helped me strike a balance between delivering technical information and making it digestible for you, my reader.

Thank you to Michelle for being my rehabilitation model as well as a star client!

Thank you Scott Sturgis for shooting the rehabilitation video for me.

Thank you to Martin Huber and Meghan Shoemaker for the illuminating medical illustrations.

Thank you to John Fellows for a fantastic design and layout.

Thank you to all my patients and clients who unwittingly served as my guinea pigs and those who wittingly modeled for pictures!

Lastly, thank you to my family for putting up with long hours of writing, meetings and physical therapy speak.

This is dedicated to my family and friends

CONTENTS

DISCLAIMER

The information contained in this book is intended to provide helpful and informative material on the subject addressed. It is not intended to serve as a replacement for professional medical advice. Any use of the information in this book is at the reader's discretion. The author and publisher specifically disclaim any and all liability arising directly or indirectly from the use or application of any information contained in this book. A health care professional should be consulted regarding your specific situation.

PREFACE

I had finished this, my sixth and final book in the Fixing You® series, long ago. But for some reason, I just wasn't happy with the information. Then I read the book *Born to Run: A Hidden Tribe, Superathletes, and the Greatest Race the World Has Never Seen* (Knopf, 2009) by Christopher McDougall. In this fascinating and entertaining read, McDougall makes a good argument that we as humans are uniquely designed to be endurance runners.

I thought, if we were designed to be endurance runners, our anatomy should reflect this. So I looked at the foot and ankle information I had put together from a different perspective, that of the requirement of walking or running tens of miles (and even hundreds!) at a time. I realized what had been nagging me: the information didn't make sense from a functional standpoint.

All my other books have shown the connection between anatomy, movement habits, and pain. Their information is based on research by Dr. Shirley Sahrmann that is featured in her seminal book, *Diagnosis and Treatment of Movement Impairment Syndromes* (Mosby, 2002). Unfortunately, this text didn't venture below the knee. Feeling like I had landed in uncharted waters, I referred back to my notes from physical therapy school as well as my research on current concepts in foot and ankle rehabilitation to serve as my guide for this last book. The problem was, when I began to look at the foot and ankle from an endurance design model, the prevailing information didn't add up.

So I threw it out and began to think: If anatomy drives function, and our anatomy seems to indicate that a certain type of function should occur, then restoring that function should eliminate foot and ankle pain. I then set out to test my ideas of what our foot and ankle anatomy means and how we should use it.

My first patient was a woman who had chronic plantar fasciitis for years. Based on my ideas of how the foot should function, I changed her foot-strike pattern and within a week it was 75% better. I was amazed! Unfortunately, she didn't achieve 100% relief because I still hadn't worked out the other systems that influence the foot. But I knew I was on the right path because each person I saw who complained of pain from plantar fasciitis, bunions, heel spurs, or shin splints reacted similarly to my recommendations.

I quickly realized, though, that people with chronic foot issues were in a deep hole in terms of function. And the first thing you do when you find yourself in a hole is stop digging. Changing people's foot-strike patterns helped do that. But that wasn't enough. They needed to be pulled out of the hole as well. That's where the other stressors to the foot and ankle come in. Once I discovered these and learned how to correct them, I began to see better results.

So I've spent the last two years testing and tweaking my theories on foot pain and what should eliminate it. As I continued my research, I began to link this information to treat back, hip, and knee pain and other areas of dysfunction.

At the same time, I've also been exploring the role of the brain in chronic pain. I've found some powerful approaches that have dramatically helped my clients with foot and ankle pain (as well as pain in other areas). These approaches are explained in Chapter 1: Mindful Healing. Essentially, I believe there is a, as yet, little understood aspect to fixing chronic pain in the body. Our brains seem to be at the heart of it. I'm continuing to experiment with integrating my limited understanding of the brain's influence on our musculoskeletal system into an efficient rehabilitation model.

I'd like to include a disclaimer though. Unlike my previous books, there is very little research supporting my claims in this book. Many health-care providers will discount this information due to a lack of studies supporting it. I can understand this. I also am doubtful of claims made without research to back them. I like to think of research as a guide to treating chronic pain though, rather than defining that treatment delivery. When research doesn't seem to provide adequate solutions to my patients' pain I must consider alternatives. This experimentation has led to this book.

Fixing You®: Foot & Ankle Pain represents my understanding to date. I can promise you that I have much more to learn! But this is a solid beginning to help you understand and fix your pain. I wish you success in your search for your answers!

INTRODUCTION

Thirty spokes converge upon a single hub,
It is on the hole in the center that the use
of the cart hinges.

We make a vessel from a lump of clay,
It is the empty space within that vessel
That makes it useful.

We make doors and windows for a room,
But it is these empty spaces that make
The room livable.

Thus, while the tangible has advantages,
It is the intangible that makes it useful.

Lao Tzu

Fixing injuries requires, among other things, an understanding of anatomy and biomechanics. That is why this book and the others in my Fixing You series presents the Fixing You approach using clear and easy-to-follow language, case studies from my practice, and pictures and diagrams to guide you, the reader, in fixing your pain. My goal is to help you visualize exactly how your body works and what is going wrong when you experience pain. When you understand and can see clearly what causes your pain, you can develop and implement a plan to fix it using the exercises and tips outlined in the Fixing You series. But knowledge is only half the answer to the problem of chronic pain. True healing also requires adjusting your mental processes to work for you, not against you.

Attention to your body and how it is or isn't working is absolutely necessary to recover from chronic pain. In fact, lack of attention is a common factor in most peoples' health issues. Developing body awareness is often the most difficult—and most important—aspect of healing from chronic pain.

Intention is another intangible but crucial aspect of healing. Harnessing your intention—your singular focus toward getting better—will reap enormous dividends. Visualize it, verbalize it, write it down, and live as if you are getting better every day; in the process you will discover which habits are counter to your goals. Once you identify these habits, you can change them. Each change will reinforce your intention. The Fixing You series presents you with knowledge about the anatomy and biomechanics of injuries, and your attention and intention makes that information useful.

A New Perspective

Since graduating from physical therapy school in 1996, I've spent hundreds of hours in continuing education classes and read countless professional journal articles and books that all attempted to answer these questions: Why do we have pain, and how do we fix it? I quickly realized there was more to injuries and healing than what I was taught in the courses I had been taking, although each had a piece of the puzzle. I realized that I needed a more complete understanding not only of how muscles and bones worked, but how they worked together to create movement.

Throughout my early years as a physical therapist, I tried one person's approach here and another's technique there. These various ideas about how to treat pain sometimes worked temporarily, but usually my clients didn't present or respond exactly like the case studies in the courses. Wanting to help people and not having the answers was frustrating. So I resolved to observe my patients closely, and I started to see the following patterns emerge:

- Patients resolving back pain using methods counter to traditional approaches.
- Chronic hamstring tightness and strains in athletes with strong hamstrings.
- Correcting structural issues in people with chronic neck pain and headaches only to have them return again and again.
- Knee pain in people whose leg muscles were strong and had good range of motion.
- Repeated straining of shoulder muscles in athletes whose musculature was strong.

In the meantime, I began exploring personal training over several years while working at an exclusive fitness club in Denver, Colorado. I had exercised all my life and found my work as a physical therapist limiting in terms of my career or life goals. Personal training seemed to be a natural extension of my interests in working with people within a larger spectrum than just treating them in a clinic.

My first client was a woman who was unable to raise her arm over her head. I reviewed her workout and found that she was doing all the wrong exercises for someone with her issues.

"Doesn't this workout hurt you?" I asked her.

"Of course it does," she replied. "Isn't it supposed to be painful?"

"No, it should be pain free," I said.

"What about 'no pain, no gain'?" she asked.

"No pain, no gain" is much like Nike's slogan "Just Do It"—you must understand that you still have to check yourself to be sure what you are doing is not harmful.

Working as a personal trainer gave me access to a type of injury that I hadn't much experience with—chronic pain. As a physical therapist in a sports and orthopedic clinic, the majority of my patients had acute injuries or surgical repairs. But there are thousands of people—if not millions—in the clubs and corporations across the United States who are exercising or working in pain, fighting chronic injuries that they've been dealing with for years, and trying to make themselves better. I know because I quickly became the busiest and highest-producing trainer/therapist at the club during my tenure there. At the time, and even now to a large extent, most people do not have access to physical therapists' musculoskeletal expertise. I was seen as something of a novelty. Thus began my quest to synthesize a more complete understanding of how dysfunction and injuries were related.

A Breakthrough

While treating one of these people, Debbie, I had an epiphany. Debbie had a 15-year history of neck pain and migraines after two back-to-back motor vehicle accidents, and she had tried everything and everyone to find relief. After a few sessions, I realized that her problem did not lie in her neck, but in her shoulder. I had made a critical connection that I previously hadn't thought about before: the structural damage the accidents had created wasn't the cause of her pain; it was caused by dysfunctional biomechanics that created vulnerabilities and which the accidents had exacerbated. We addressed these functional issues, and within a few days her pain had disappeared.

Just as I was finishing with Debbie, I discovered a book that confirmed my diagnosis and treatment approach with her as well as a few of my other chronic pain patients. Written by Dr. Shirley A. Sahrmann, a physical therapist out of Washington University in St. Louis, *Diagnosis and Treatment of Movement Impairment Syndromes* is a medical textbook that provided the missing link I had been seeking to pull together my observations. Many of the biomechanical paradigms and rehabilitative exercises in the Fixing You series have been adapted from Dr. Sahrmann's brilliant textbook. I recommend that all physical therapists purchase the book and attend her courses.

Another book I regularly reference is Florence Kendall, Elizabeth McCreary, and Patricia Provance's classic, *Muscles Testing and Function:with posture and pain.* This textbook is a wealth of information for understanding precise musculoskeletal anatomy and testing. It is a standard in physical therapy, and I regularly refer to it for isolating muscle testing. It guides me in specifically analyzing and thinking creatively about function. By understanding muscle function on a basic level, I can better hypothesize functional deficits that may be occurring at a systemic level.

Lastly I need to mention Dr. Thomas Hanna who developed Hanna Somatics. He wrote *Somatics: reawakening the mind's control of movement, flexibility, and health,* and has been instrumental in introducing me to the brain's role in working with chronic pain. His unique books and courses have helped me integrate biomechanics into patterns of movement. This has helped me see the body more as a whole, rather than a series of parts.

But my books are written for laypeople, not medical professionals, to guide you in healing yourself. I've simplified and distilled my medical training to reflect the majority of problems I've found when treating clients. I've prioritized the corrective exercises I've found most powerful for most conditions. I've bolded vocabulary words and added information boxes to help clarify words or concepts. I've also created videos of all the exercises and tests to enhance the effectiveness of your program. To access these free video clips, visit my website **www.FixingYou.net**. Type in the code at the end of this book (pg 100) to access the extra material.

Holistic Function

The body is the sum of individual units working together to create functional movement. Bones, muscles, tendons, nerves, and ligaments can all be addressed individually, but it is important to understand how these structures work collectively with the brain to fulfill a purpose: pain-free movement of the body. So, while it is imperative that individual "chinks in the armor" are found and corrected, visualizing how the whole works together is just as important. This concept also works from the other direction; training movement and/or function reinforces and assists in correcting individual muscles' poor performance. In this book, I've introduced the key individual players—the parts that make up the whole—and also shown how they play together to create function, much like a symphony. You are responsible for bringing them in line to create your concert.

I wish you the best in your pursuit for solutions to your pain. You are not alone in your search for answers. I truly believe that, with a little thought and effort on your part, the Fixing You approach will help you find your answers, as it has for my clients.

The beauty of the body is that results happen quickly when you are doing the right thing. Most of the clients you will read about, and those that aren't included in this book, feel significantly better after only one or two treatments. Often, my clients understand they are on the right path within minutes of performing an exercise. Emboldened by this sense, they become more committed to the process of fixing themselves. You can have the same feeling of empowerment. There is no magical technique or device that will fix you. Only you can fix you—so let's get started on giving you the tools to do just that.

1 | Mindful Healing

There is not a single problem in life
*you cannot **resolve**, provided you first*
*solve it in your **inner world**,*
its place of origin.

—Paramahansa Yogananda

Time and time again I see clients who have tried so many unsuccessful cures that they just don't know what to do. This is worrisome—not because I believe they can't be helped, but because *they* don't believe they can be helped.

The most powerful aspect of the Fixing You® approach is that it shows you what is wrong, actually getting you to feel or sense that certain muscles or movements are not working and how your pain changes when they are corrected. This helps define the problem. It gives issues a beginning and an end, allowing you to compartmentalize pain and therefore see when and how the solution will happen.

Given the tools to understand and correct your injuries, I hope you will feel a sense of empowerment that will motivate you to work harder to fix yourself. If you can define an injury, then you have the power to fix it—and that motivation will get you results.

Defining an injury (especially if it is a chronic problem) is more than just understanding the muscles and bones involved. It's understanding how and why those muscles and bones are behaving like they are. They just don't move (or not move) or become tight (or loose) on their own. Everything they do is controlled in some way by your brain. Your brain is actually telling your body to behave in a way that is causing you pain. Once you can understand this and control how the brain is delivering these messages and what it takes to change the brain's instructions, you'll be well on your way to fixing your problems. It may be a challenge for you to discover this deep-seated neural programming. Nevertheless it must be replaced with better programming to fully heal your body. This is what empowerment is all about—giving yourself the power to change your brain, your body, and your life. It's not just a nice concept; it is actually something you can harness. But in order to harness it, you need to know a little more about how your brain and body work together. The following information will hopefully give you insight into some unseen but important players involved with your pain.

Fascia, the brain, and pain

Fascia

If you've ever heard the expression "You can't see the forest for the trees," then you'll have an appreciation for the presence of **fascia** in our bodies. Fascia is connective tissue that blends into, wraps around, or connects every structure in the body. Often in anatomy dissections, the difficult part of teasing out different muscles, nerves, blood vessels, or organs is separating them from all the fascia that surrounds and binds them. Because of this, fascia has often been overlooked and instead seen as a nuisance that hinders dissections rather than being appreciated for its structural support of the musculoskeletal system.

> **Fascia** is a continuous network of connective tissue that wraps around just about everything in the body. Because of this, **problems in one area** can translate into pain in a remote location.

There are many different kinds of fascia. For example, a spider-web-like fascia connects our skin to our muscles and muscles to muscles; we also have thick fascial sheaths like fabric that connect structures in our body. An example of this is the tough sheet of plantar fascia on the bottoms of our feet. The important thing to remember is that fascia connects to, supports, disperses tension from, and delivers tension to every structure in the body. Because it invests in all of our muscles, bones, and nerves and has varying thicknesses, it can be seen as continuous tissue. For instance, it turns out that various strong lines of fascia connect our toes to our head (Figure 1.1).[1] Figure 1.1 depicts one of these lines traveling throughout our body.[2] These tension pathways include muscles, tendons, and ligaments and help distribute force away from sites of trauma. Looking at this picture, you can imagine how the foot may affect neck function or headaches. We are just beginning to be explore this fascinating tissue in terms of movement, and I think will become an ever-growing factor in our pursuit of understanding chronic pain.

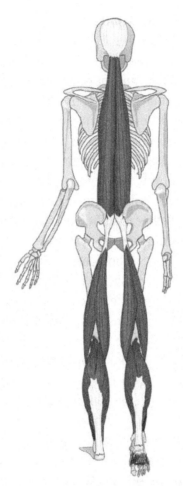

Superficial Back Line

Figure 1.1 Strong lines of fascia links bones, muscles, and nerves throughout the body.

Fascia is also rich in nerves. In fact, many of the nerves found in fascia are of a little known group—types III and IV. These nerves are considered **mechanoreceptors**, which means they respond to mechanical tension or pressure.[3] They also may respond to pain, which can then increase their sensitivity to changes in tension or pressure. Fascia is also invested with a type of smooth muscle.[4] Smooth muscle is different than skeletal muscle in that it is considered to be involuntary (we can't make it contract) and is mostly found in our viscera. Certain contractile cells that make up fascia, **myofibroblasts**, are sensitive to chemical changes rather than neural changes. In other words, unlike our skeletal muscles which respond to messages traveling through our nerves, these smooth muscles within the fascia respond to chemicals in their midst. It has yet to be determined exactly which chemicals stimulate contraction of these smooth muscles.

The idea here is that tension can be generated within the fascial system. Because fascia connects to everything in our bodies and is especially invested in muscles, tendons, ligaments, and bones, this ability to create tension may help explain connections of pain in one area of the body to movement dysfunction in other areas.

We have much to learn about this hidden forest in our bodies. We are just beginning to turn our focus to this overlooked and fascinating network within us. I'm confident that future research and clinical studies will prove this system is integral to our movement health.

> **A fibroblast** is a cell that makes collagen, a principle component of fascia. **Myofibroblasts** are fibroblasts that are also capable of contraction similar to that found in smooth muscle.

Client Connection

Recently I saw a woman with plantar fasciitis and sciatic pain in the same leg. After working together and resolving her pain, at the end of the session she realized that the headache she'd had for the last three days had also disappeared. We only worked on her lower extremities, but I believe that what we actually did was relieve stress along the Superficial Back Line (Figure 1.1), which connects her feet to the top of her head. I'm just beginning to experiment with fascial connections in our body, but there are therapists who've been studying these systems for years and may be a good resource to seek out if you have chronic pain.

The Brain

If I asked you to lift your leg, you'd just lift it, almost without a thought. It's a movement you've performed millions of times in your life. In fact, go ahead and try it now while you're sitting down. Lift one of your legs off the ground about 2 or 3 inches and then lower it back down. Do you notice something different about how that leg feels now? Just a minute ago, you probably weren't even aware of your leg, but now that I've asked you to move it you might, on some level, sense it more. You may have realized that it wasn't completely relaxed before, but now that you've paid attention, it may feel heavier and more relaxed than your other leg. Or maybe you've just become aware of the fact that you can't seem to relax it fully.

You've just tapped into the most sophisticated movement system on Earth. Front and center is your brain, about which we still have so much to learn. The brain connects to the spine, and out of the spine runs a vast network of nerves that make it possible to sense and move your leg. These nerves invest bone, muscles, fascia, blood vessels—basically everything in your body.

Your brain and body have a complicated feedback system to make sure you lifted that leg up instead of pushed it down, that it lifted smoothly rather than in an abrupt jerk, and that your foot didn't kick out at the same time the leg was moving. A myriad of communications that you were unaware of occurred to and from your brain to fine tune that simple leg lift. We really make movement look easy!

But sometimes things don't go so smoothly—especially when there is trauma to a region. Trauma can occur as a result of an accident, or it can be gradual, slowly building due to deeply ingrained movement habits or other causes such as emotional or psychological events. Unknown to you, your brain makes adjustments to how it maintains muscles' length and tension in response to these traumas. Usually this is in the form of developing tension in the muscles and fascia.

The following idea is at the root of most chronic pain: *Your body is harboring unconscious contractions ultimately exerting excessive tension through tissues and joints.*

Yes, you may be able to stretch those muscles through their full ranges of motion, but they will usually return to the contracted length because that is where your brain thinks it needs to hold them to avoid pain. Your brain doesn't know that it can allow those muscles to lengthen and remain lengthened.

This is the idea behind one approach to fixing your pain—becoming aware of your areas of trauma and problem muscles and then learning to lengthen and relax them, both psychologically and physically. The key to this lies in how our brain works, so bear with me while I introduce the two of you.

Our ability to sense and move our muscles is found in our brain. This can get pretty complicated, but the **sensorimotor cortex** is integral to this process. The sensorimotor cortex is a region of the brain that runs through the center and spans both halves (Figure 1.2).

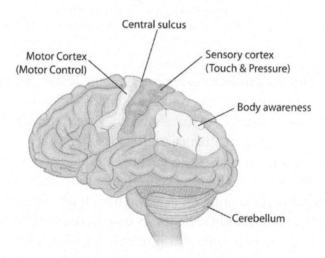

The Sensorimotor Cortex

Figure 1.2 The sensorimotor cortex is important in sensing and moving our bodies.

The sensory portion of the brain, also referred to as the somatosensory cortex, receives messages from our muscles; information from our senses like pressure or touch. Our body is mapped onto the sensory cortex with the most-used parts taking up more space in the brain. This map can be represented as a **homunculus** (Figure 1.3).

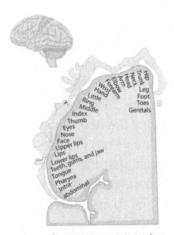

Somatosensory cortex in
right cerebral hemisphere

The Sensory Homunculus

Figure 1.3 The sensory homunculus represents proportionally how
our sensing body is m apped on our brain.

The **voluntary motor cortex** is the motor or movement portion of the sensorimotor cortex. We have a motor cortex homunculus too, which looks similar to the sensory cortex homunculus (Figure 1.4). Notice how the hands and areas of the face are larger. We have more brain real estate devoted to these senses and motions than the rest of the body because they are so important to us: the hands for manipulating objects and mouth for communication.

Your brain constantly changes its map in response to how you use your body. If you look at a professional violinist's homunculus, you might find more area devoted to the hands and fingers than the average person's because violinists use extreme fine motor coordination in their work. The brain adapts by increasing the real estate this area uses frequently. Likewise, parts of the body that aren't used as much may result in a shrinkage of the real estate that controls that region.

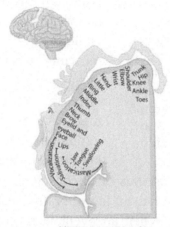

Motor cortex in right
cerebral hemisphere

The Motor Homunculus

Figure 1.4 The motor homunculus represents proportionally how
our moving body is mapped on our brain.

The body responds to what the brain tells it to do. So when you put your hand on some gooey gum at a baseball game, the nerves in your skin send a signal to your sensory cortex saying "Yuck, my hand is in something sticky!" Your motor cortex, right next door, quickly sends a message along your nerves to get your hand out of that gum ASAP! That's basically how the body, or really the brain, works: it senses and negotiates our environment. Sometimes this is reflexive or automatic, and sometimes we plan our movement.

Okay, that's all fairly straightforward, but why did I go through all that neurology? *Because one of the keys to changing unconscious tension or contraction of your muscles, and therefore pain, will be to sense it.* The brain must understand what it is dealing with before it can change what is happening. This is just as important with psychological or emotional tension as with muscular tension. In fact, it is often difficult to separate the two.

Although the exact pathways are not clear, we understand that psychological stress contributes to muscular tension. Hardly a week goes by that I don't hear someone say they carry their stress in their neck or back. Each of us has a unique history, and our brains house all those memories and experiences, whether conscious or unconscious. The events we have experienced are mapped out in our brains, just as our sensory and motor cortices are. When an event is stressful enough, or that stress remains over an extended time, our physical body adapts to it through muscular contraction or through changes to our lymphatic system, which fights off disease.[5] Over time this influences how we move and live our lives, which establishes neural pathways of movement that eventually break down our physical systems and cause pain or sickness.

Want to learn more about the brain? I highly recommend the entertaining and informative book **The Brain that Changes Itself: Stories of Personal Triumph from the Frontiers of Brain Science** by Norman Doidge.

Emotional stressors that I often run into with my patients are anger, fear, and frustration. Anger and frustration often arise because many patients I see have been through a host of doctors and specialists trying to find answers. These emotions can't be directed to a specific person and so are held internally. Often our society doesn't allow us to express this anger, or we have been taught that anger is bad and therefore shouldn't be expressed, so the patient is left holding the bag, so to speak. Anger or frustration could be due to secondary fallout from the chronic pain—medical bills, loss of employment, or loss of quality family time, just to name a few. Or the anger and frustration could be a preexisting issue that has manifested as pain. Regardless, it must be acknowledged and resolved in some way to help heal the physical manifestation of it. You've heard the saying "Laughter is the best medicine." Well, in terms of stress and pain, it often can be a huge help.

Client Connection

A while ago a man came to see me for neck pain. I couldn't find anything wrong with him but gave him a couple of exercises designed to relieve stress to the neck region. He seemed irritated that he had to do these exercises. He came back a week later, clearly agitated, and stated his neck pain had not changed. So we sat down, and I told him that I couldn't find anything physically wrong with his neck. I also told him that people didn't typically speak to me in the tone or manner he was using, and I believed he had some anger issues that he needed to address. He said of course he was angry—his neck hurt! He was only able to come in on Thursdays, and I told him I wouldn't be able to see him the following week because it was Thanksgiving. He responded sarcastically, "Great, Thanksgiving!" So I reflected his emotions back to him and said, "Yeah, Thanksgiving. What a bummer!" He looked at me stunned and after a few moments said, "Geez, I really do have an anger problem don't I? How could I be angry about Thanksgiving?" I told him I thought he did and this may be why he had neck pain. I asked him to see a counselor or therapist about it to get at the roots of the problem. He called the following week to say his neck pain was completely gone after addressing his anger issues.

I often hear fear in the statements of my chronic pain patients too—fear that they will not get better, fear that they have become vulnerable, fear that they may hurt themselves further, or fear that they'll never live their lives again. This fear can immobilize people and should be discussed with a therapist. Often the message played in a patient's mind is a self-destructive loop such as "I'll never be able to do X again because of my pain." This is a self-fulfilling prophecy for many because their fear prevents them from exploring solutions. Which means they probably won't resolve their pain and get to do X again.

Often this fear is well-founded because many people are told that exercise is the key to eliminating pain. However, when they've tried to exercise, their pain has gotten worse. If a person doesn't understand why or how their movement patterns are contributing to their pain in the first place, exercise can often magnify the problem by adding more repetition or load to the vulnerable system and tissues. So they fear more exercise because they've learned that doesn't help and may have even hurt them more. This fear also introduces more tension to our body-brain systems, which propagates the pain cycle.

Client Connection

One of my very first clients as a recently graduated physical therapist was a woman whose lips, fingertips, and toes turned blue with exertion. This began after her husband had a heart attack and was in the hospital three months prior to our meeting. After she visited him, she went home and cleaned the house from top to bottom. The next morning she woke up with blue fingertips. She went through a lot of testing, and no one seemed to have a clue as to what was going on with her. Neither did I.

During our second appointment, after failing to help her in our first session, I sat down with her and reviewed her history.

"Iris, your husband had a heart attack three months ago," I began. She nodded, looking concerned.

"How's he doing?"

"He's much better. He's just started a walking program." She brightened a little.

Then what I needed to say next came to me. I looked her straight in the eyes and said, "Iris, your husband isn't going to die." She blinked. "And neither are you," I continued. She blinked again and let out a deep sigh.

I felt I was onto the source of her problem and continued, "Have you ever spoken of this to a therapist, counselor, priest, or friend? Anyone who you can confide in?"

"No, I haven't," she said.

"Then your treatment is to do so within the next four days. I'll see you in a week," I finished.

She came back next week, arm-in-arm with her husband and looking radiant. She had spoken to a therapist and was completely symptom free. Her blood vessels were no longer constricting from her fear of her or her husband's death.

Acknowledging fears and speaking to a trained therapist will help a patient truly understand its place in their lives. I am not a trained psychologist and recommend my patients to these services if I believe there is an element of psychological stress contributing to their pain (which is often the case if pain has become chronic or no one seems to understand the causes). It's unfortunate that many people feel there is a stigma associated with seeing a therapist and insist instead that their problems are entirely physical. Even if they are, it wouldn't hurt to explore this connection between the mind and the body. If a therapist is not available, writing about your emotions or stress in a journal can often be of great help too. The idea is to get the issues out in the open so you can see them and therefore resolve them. Remember, the brain can't fix what it can't sense.

To that end, I am including a Schedule of Life Events developed by Dr. Thomas Holmes and fellow researchers at the University of Washington School of Medicine.[6] He and his team found that higher levels of stress in our lives correlated to higher chances of illness. They came up with a way to quantify this relationship. I believe this also extends to musculoskeletal problems. This schedule, together with instructions about how to fill it out and evaluate stress in your life, can be found in Appendix A in the back of this book.

From a physical perspective, in response to these emotional or physical traumas and unknown to you, your brain signals your muscles to reflexively contract. Somehow we must help your brain sense what is happening and educate it to allow these muscles to move through their full ranges of motion or learn to rest them fully.

Try this little test: bend and straighten your elbow two or three times. You've just used your biceps muscles on the front upper part of your arm to bend that elbow and lower it down again. But did you feel the biceps muscles working? Most of you would probably answer no, you just bent and straightened your arm. This is how most of us move and work from day to day: we do it, but are unaware of what is really happening.

This time apply a couple pounds of resistance to the muscles by pressing gently against your wrist, as if taking your pulse. Now bend and slowly straighten the elbow all the way down, maintaining that light resistance. Do you feel your biceps muscles now? If not, increase the resistance until you do.

> Releasing a muscle involves contracting and then slowly lengthening it while providing a little resistance. This helps remove reflexive or unconscious contraction of that muscle to restore it to its normal resting length and tension.

You've just connected your brain to your biceps muscles by using a little resistance against them so your brain could actually sense the length and tension of your muscles while straightening your arm. Once you remove the resistance and allow your arm to rest, you may experience more awareness of those biceps muscles. You may also notice that you can rest them more deeply. This latter observation comes from the fact that your brain now has a clearer idea of how much contraction is needed to maintain the length and tension of those muscles when they aren't in use— which is very little. I'll refer to the idea of improving the resting length and tension of a muscle as "releasing the muscle."

This treatment protocol, helping your brain reestablish an ideal tension-length relationship of your muscles, is at the core of Hanna Somatics, developed by Dr. Thomas Hanna. Dr. Hanna identified three reflexive patterns in the body contributing to chronic pain. According to him, these three patterns are at the root of most chronic pain and can occur simultaneously in different areas of the body. He found that systematically releasing these muscles, through contraction and slow lengthening, corrected many of these reflexive patterns and eliminated pain.

Releasing a muscle is different than stretching a muscle. Let's go back to your biceps muscle. The brain has determined that it is comfortable maintaining a certain contracted length and tension of that muscle so it can better sense it and therefore keep it ready to do work if necessary. If we stretch it, your

> Two interesting books written by Dr. Thomas Hanna are **Somatics: Reawakening the Mind's Control of Movement, Flexibility, and Health;** and **The Body of Life: Creating New Pathways for Sensory Awareness and Fluid Movement.**

brain will think that's nice, but it will return the muscle to the length and tension it has previously been taught are appropriate because it hasn't learned anything new about that muscle. So you will have to stretch it again and again for a long time, and rest and use it in that lengthened position, before your brain and body adapt to allow this new length.

> An **eccentric contraction** allows the muscle to lengthen while contracting the muscle at the same time.

Releasing the muscle is different because the muscle remains gently contracted while slowly lengthening. This uses a controlled **eccentric contraction** that the brain can more easily sense. Reflexive contractions are minimized during this process because, as the brain maintains sense of the contracted muscle, it is in control of this lengthening process rather than being overridden by excessive force, as with stretching. This resets the resting length of the muscle because the brain will have learned that it can maintain the same tension but with the muscle now lengthened. Stretching the muscle doesn't teach this to the brain.

This may not seem like a big deal now because you don't have pain in your biceps muscles, but applying this strategy to painful chronically contracted muscles can eliminate your pain entirely by freeing the muscles to lengthen through their complete ranges of motion without any reflexive return to a contracted state (that is, if the sources of those contracted states are resolved, such as with emotional stress or movement dysfunctions). This restores normal joint range of motion and freedom of movement, and it reduces tension across the joint. I also believe this changes the tension of various lines of fascia running through our bodies (like the Superficial Back Line mentioned earlier in this chapter). Because fascia and muscles are so closely intertwined, I believe one affects the other.

As I mentioned earlier, most pain is caused by chronically contracted muscles changing how joints function, which then reinforces the contracted muscles. Therefore several of the exercises I recommend in this book will employ this strategy of releasing muscles. In a nutshell, this involves providing gentle resistance to a muscle group while sensing and lengthening that group. In most cases you will need someone else to help you to get the best results.

A Stranger to Yourself

Another idea to keep in mind while fixing yourself is that sometimes you will have to be an observer of your own body in order to correct your movement habits. To illustrate this, quickly interlace your fingers as if praying. You probably didn't even have to look at your hands to do this. Now look down to see which thumb is on top. Left or right? Look at the rest of your fingers and note which hand's fingers are on top of the others. You probably didn't even know you would lace your fingers like that, did you? Now undo the fingers and quickly interlace them with the other hand's fingers and thumb on top. I bet you had to look at your hands in order to do this. One or two fingers may have stumbled and you had to work out where they needed to go. You may have needed to look closely at your results to make sure each finger actually went to the right spot. Holding this new position probably feels very foreign to you, and you may even make the judgment that this position is "wrong" or "bad" as compared to your preferred method of interlacing the fingers.

This is what I mean by becoming an observer of your own body. Sometimes, in order to learn a new way of doing things, you need to watch your body to make sure it is doing something right. Because the brain wants to use established patterns of movement, it will try to override these new movement patterns *even though they may eliminate your pain.* So just be aware that although your new movements may not feel natural, it doesn't mean they are harmful. In fact, the opposite may be true; your natural movements may actually be harmful.

Another aspect of creating new movement habits is to visualize them. Visualization has gained greater acceptance in the field of athletic performance because visualizing particular movements activates the circuitry in your brain that will be used when actually performing those movements. Rehearsing ideal movement in your mind begins the changes that will need to take place to completely retrain your movement habits. Then, once you begin changing your habits, the neural pathways you use will become more quickly engrained—much like forging a new hiking trail. The first time you do it, it will require more energy, but as the trail becomes more used, it will be easier to hike on it. To do this you must also be able to sense when you are doing something harmful. That's where the next chapter comes in.

The muscle-releasing exercises I offer in this book will ask you to follow a similar

Sensory input/feedback + motor control = optimal muscle efficiency

The converse is also true: optimal muscle efficiency is degraded by loss of sensory input and/or motor control.

pattern, that of gently contracting and slowly releasing muscles through their full ranges of motion while focusing on the muscles you are affecting. Your awareness (sensory input to the sensory cortex) is crucial to maintain control of the muscles (via the voluntary motor cortex) and therefore their complete release (restoration of an improved length and tension relationship).This will be reinforced by using those muscles differently. I've included images of most muscles to help you visualize where they begin and end to help you maintain your awareness while you release them.

Especially for the foot and lower leg muscles, I highly recommend you watch the video clips of these exercises to understand the nuances of these techniques. They can be accessed by going to the "Foot and Ankle" page of the Fixing You® website and typing in the code found on page 100 in the back of this book.

A last word on stretching. You might think, based on this information, that I'm against stretching. I'm not. I think stretching offers a good short-term benefit to gaining muscle length. What I'm advocating is an alternative, long-term solution to your pain. Often the results are just as quick if not more so. But old habits (and beliefs) die hard, so continue with your stretching routine if you believe it is helping you. Sometimes it's worth stretching simply because it feels good!

So, if we think about why we have chronic pain we might think of it as a cycle or loop of problems feeding each other. That cycle might look like this.

The brain is the sensing and directing organ of all our experiences. Whether it is physical, visual, aural (hearing), emotional (via stress or trauma), olfactorial (smelling), or lingual (taste), this information enters our brain. The processing of this information involves intricate neural pathways connecting different areas of the brain and may trigger a motor response (muscular contraction), whether conscious or unconscious. This motor response involves our muscular and fascial (myofascial) systems, which affect how we rest and move. Preferred resting or movement patterns (biomechanics) become engrained neural pathways that are learned and reinforced by the brain. The brain continues using these movement patterns, which become deeply entrenched through repetition, and the cycle continues reinforcing itself (Figure 1.5).

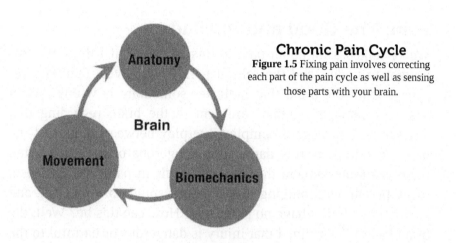

Chronic Pain Cycle
Figure 1.5 Fixing pain involves correcting each part of the pain cycle as well as sensing those parts with your brain.

However, from a tissue perspective, these movement patterns may be delivering local stress to joints or other tissues, injuring them. Perhaps the brain will sense these local stresses and unconsciously avoid them by creating alternative patterns that may stress other tissues in the process. Or the brain may ignore these stresses entirely because we are consciously overriding new movement patterns due to the influence of a particular goal (such as a work quota, athletic performance goals, ergonomic constraints, and so on). It will be helpful to keep this image in your mind while working through your issues to remind you that several systems are involved in movement, any one (or several) of which can create pain.

Sometimes the problems and solutions are purely biomechanical. These can be corrected through changing movement patterns, lengthening muscles, strengthening weaknesses, or other physical means. Other times there is an emotional component that also generates tension within the musculoskeletal system and manifests in certain holding/movement patterns. These issues must be addressed to help eliminate chronic pain. Quite frequently both of these scenarios are playing out to some degree in difficult cases of chronic pain.

Pain: The Good and the Bad

We've talked a lot about pain in this chapter, but I think it's important to understand the role of pain in our lives. Pain is a response from the brain that indicates something is wrong. When tissue is damaged, signals are sent to the brain regarding that damage and, through a complex interplay between centers of the brain, it interprets this damage as dangerous or harmful. Often there is tissue damage that doesn't result in pain. For instance, many people with bulging disks in their spine, torn menisci, and even broken bones have no pain at all. How can this be? Well, the brain hasn't determined that injury is dangerous or harmful to the overall function of the body in that particular person.

Pain, then, is something we experience that tells us something is wrong with us. It would be really nice if we had a computer we could plug ourselves into, similar to a car diagnostic computer, that spits out the exact problem. Unfortunately, we don't; that is where medical professionals come in. But because the human body is so complex (much more so than a car) and we understand so little about how our magnificent machines actually work, there are many different approaches to looking at our function. I liken it to the story about the five blind men, all touching a different part of an elephant and determining what that elephant is based on their experience. The first blind man, feeling the elephant's trunk, thinks the elephant is a big, thick, strong tube that can grip things. The second blind

> **Explain Pain** by David S. Butler and G. Lorimer Moseley is a great book to more thoroughly understand the hows and whys of pain.

man, feeling the elephant's ears, believes the elephant is like a big, floppy, thin leaf. The third blind man, feeling the elephant's tummy, describes the elephant as a big barrel. The fourth, feeling the elephant's legs, thinks the elephant is like a tree trunk. And the fifth blind man, feeling the elephant's tail, thinks the elephant is like a small snake.

None of them are wrong, yet all of them are wrong. Until we can fully understand how all systems of the body work together, we are like the blind men describing the elephant. This is why there are so many perspectives about why you have pain. As a patient, you must think critically about the information you're receiving. Does it make sense? Does it explain why you are having pain? In the case of back pain, did that disc bulge just appear the day before you experienced your pain or has it been there for a while and suddenly resulted in pain? If it's been there for a while, then why didn't you experience pain before? If it just appeared, then why? Do disc bulges develop in a day? My belief is that, ultimately, you must fix yourself; you must take responsibility for your health and ask these questions. I personally love it when people challenge me. These are the people who usually get better quickly, and they keep me on my toes to make sure I'm considering everything. The patient and I are partners in their healing rather than me being a dictator.

So, getting back to pain, let's look at it a little more closely. It is a natural reaction to avoid a stimulus that is hurting you. The operative premise here is that it is hurting you. Quite often I need to educate my clients regarding "good" pain versus "bad" pain. The discomfort of a fatigued muscle feels different than the pain of a muscle strain or impinged joint—pain that indicates injury. Learning to tell the difference between "good" pain (the temporary discomfort of retraining your body) and "bad" pain (pain that indicates injury) is important to your healing process.

Generally, what I'm referring to as "good" pain is a feeling of fatigue in the muscles or tissues you are exercising or trying to restore range of motion to. Muscle fatigue may be uncomfortable, but it doesn't mean that what we're doing is hurting us; in fact, that feeling of fatigue lets us know that we are getting stronger. Muscle fatigue also indicates that your body has had enough for the time being. Listen to your body. Stop when you need to. Don't try to push through another set of repetitions or add more weight until your body is ready. Avoiding the message your body is sending doesn't do you any favors and ultimately slows down your progress because ignoring good pain establishes compensatory behavior that can contribute to bad pain.

For example, imagine that you are performing a biceps curl, bending your elbow to bring your hand to the top of your shoulder and then lowering it back down to your side. Weightlifters perform this exercise with weights in their hands to strengthen the biceps muscles in the front of their arms. To maintain good form during this exercise, the arm should stay roughly at the midpoint of the trunk while curling the hand up and down. This helps the head of the arm bone, nestled in the shoulder socket, remain in its proper position with limited stress to the shoulder joint tissues.

Keeping the arm in a mechanically correct position fatigues the biceps muscles more quickly and with lighter weight. However, if weightlifters push past fatigue in order to reach a predetermined number of repetitions or lift heavier weight, the elbow compensates by rocking forward and back. When the elbow moves back, the head of the arm bone at the shoulder joint moves forward, often pulling the shoulder blade with it or stressing the tissues in the front of the shoulder. Over time, this can create a host of mechanical problems in the shoulder joint or neck.

Biceps fatigue during curls is good pain because it indicates that the muscle is being stimulated to strengthen and grow. This is what we're shooting for when performing strengthening exercises. We want muscle stimulation and therefore improved strength and control of the bone or joint in question. In the biceps curl example, ignoring this fatigue to squeeze out a few more reps or allow you to lift more weight can cause shoulder joint problems. Become comfortable with and even rejoice in the fact that the muscle you are targeting is fatiguing. It is better to incrementally strengthen the muscle group rather than compensate your form—and your healing process—to squeeze out a few more repetitions. This is where bad pain comes in.

Avoidance of good pain—ignoring your body's signals—often leads to "bad" pain. Bad pain is more difficult to describe because everyone experiences it differently. It can be sharp or dull, nagging or acute. It is the pain you are trying to eliminate, the pain of injury or dysfunction. It is something you instinctively know shouldn't be happening.

You should only feel fatigue in the muscles you are targeting. Using the biceps curl example, if you feel pain at the shoulder or elbow joints while performing the curl, then you know you're experiencing bad pain. The biceps muscles are located between the shoulder and elbow joints. If you feel pain above or below the biceps muscles, it's likely that you are lifting too heavy a load or allowing your elbows to move too much. The habits that cause bad pain ultimately compromise your efforts, leading to tissue vulnerability and weakness—and more pain.

So often, clients are disappointed to find that they fatigue quickly when exercising with correct form. I happily point out that this is great news because they are finally activating and strengthening the right muscles without exacerbating their condition! Keep this in mind as you strengthen through your injury.

Attention and Awareness

Chronic aches and pains aren't just for those who have been involved in accidents. I've found similar biomechanical problems at the roots of chronic pain in people who have had traumatic accidents as well as in those who didn't. Therefore, I believe accidents expose and exacerbate existing vulnerabilities in our bodies. Working with someone who was involved in a motor vehicle accident that resulted in, say, chronic neck pain has been no different than helping someone who has had headaches and neck pain for decades and has never been involved in an accident. They both require an understanding of how poor function is feeding the problem and what needs to be corrected to eliminate pain. Essentially, in order to fix your body and eliminate chronic pain, you need to pay attention to how your body moves.

I used to work at a health club. While I was in the locker room changing after a workout one day, a man approached me.

"Hey, do you mind taking a look at my arm? I bumped it last week and now I don't seem to have strength like I used to," he said.

"Sure," I said.

In three seconds, I knew exactly what his problem was; he had completely severed his biceps tendon at the elbow. His injured arm was visibly smaller than the other arm, and the biceps muscle was curled up in a little ball up by his shoulder, similar to the way blinds roll up on windows. It was as if someone had stuffed a sock into his upper arm.

"You've ruptured your biceps tendon," I said, "and you need to get an orthopedic surgeon to operate on it immediately."

This man ended up having an emergency operation to fix his severed biceps. Needless to say, he was not in touch with his body. Many of you reading this book are in a similar situation—not ever considering how different parts of your body work together to create pain-free movement. In the above case, a man had suffered a traumatic blow to his arm that caused his problem. In this regard, it was a clear-cut issue that had an easily pinpointed cause. But chronic pain is often caused by a gradual decline in the quality of the body's movements; unfortunately, your stress levels increase the pace of this decline, which further emphasizes the problem. It is time for you to pay attention to your body, and my sincerest hope is that the information in this book will help you do that. The exercises in this book will help you if you check in with yourself and become aware of your movement habits. Always go back to your form and think about what you are doing. Be present and be attentive. You will be rewarded for it!

In summary, chronic pain can occur as a result of emotional or physical stress or trauma (prolonged or a single occurrence), habitual movement patterns, or both. The brain often responds to stress by increasing myofascial tension, which can further impair movement habits. Understanding the nature of this stress and its consequences is the first step in unraveling the mystery of chronic pain.

You will need to pay attention to your body to heal yourself. In my experience, it is a fascinating journey of discovery to learn why people do what they do to create pain. To lessen the stress involved with this endeavor, think about it as a game of hide-and-seek. Something you are doing is causing pain in your body, and it's hiding from your awareness. Now it's time for you to start methodically looking for those culprits. In the process, you'll have many Aha! moments where you'll make connections between your habits or behaviors and your pain.

I was recently working with a golfer with low back pain, and we discovered the movement pattern that caused his pain and what to do to fix it. Then I said, "Now pretend you're putting the golf tee into the ground to tee off," and he immediately reverted back to his old way of moving. This was because he had very deep neural patterns associated with golf that he hadn't yet connected to his improved pattern of movement. Putting these pieces together will eliminate his pain. I think this is fascinating. I hope you can think of it that way too!

1 Thomas Myers, *Anatomy Trains: Myofascial Meridians for Manual and Movement Therapists,* 2nd edition (Churchill Livingstone, 2008).

2 Adapted from Thomas Myers, *Anatomy Trains: Myofascial Meridians for Manual and Movement Therapists,* 2nd edition (Churchill Livingstone, 2008).0

3 Robert Schleip, "Fascial Plasticity—A New Neurobiological Explanation: Part 1," *Journal of Bodywork and Movement Therapies* 7 (1), 11–19.

4 Robert Schleip, "Fascial Plasticity—A New Neurobiological Explanation: Part 1," *Journal of Bodywork and Movement Therapies* 7 (2), 104–16.

5 Esther M. Sternberg, *The Balance Within: The Science of Connecting Health and Emotions* (W. H. Freeman, 2001), 111–12.

6 Thomas H. Holmes and Richard H. Rahe, "The Social Readjustment Rating Scale," *Journal of Psychosomatic Research* 11 (2), 213–18.

2 Understanding Your Anatomy

Knowledge *of any kind gets metabolized spontaneously and brings about a* **change** *in* **awareness** *from where it is possible to create* **new realities**.

—**Deepak Chopra**

The Bones and Movements of the Foot

An important idea to keep in mind about foot pain is that the foot doesn't work in isolation. The knee, hip, and even shoulder joint mechanics affect foot function almost as much as the mechanics within the foot. I think the best place to begin, though, is gaining a basic understanding about the bones of the foot and lower leg.

There are 26 bones in the human foot, not bad considering there are 27 in the human hand and wrist! To me that means the foot must be a pretty important, not to mention complicated, piece of real estate. You'll notice that the architecture of these bones creates an arch in the foot. The maintenance of this arch is as important to foot function as the lumbar curve is to low back function. When excessive stresses act on this arch, foot problems ensue.

You'll notice in Figure 2.1 that the **fibula** and **tibia** flank both sides of the foot to help form the ankle joint. The tibia goes on to articulate with the thigh bone (**femur**) and knee cap (**patella**) to form the knee joint. The fibula almost makes it up to the knee joint but not quite. It is anchored to the tibia by **ligaments** and a long **interosseous membrane**. As you'll see, several muscles that insert into the foot originate from this membrane.

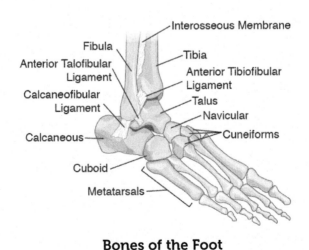

Bones of the Foot

Figure 2.1 There are 26 bones in the human foot.

At the ankle, the tibia interacts with the **talus** bone, which is ir-regularly shaped, to form the ankle joint. On the outside is the fibula. As you can see in Figure 2.1, lots of ligaments connect the bones of the foot to the fibula and tibia and also connect the fibula and tibia. These ligaments are important for ankle stability.

The shape of the talus bone dictates that the foot does not just move straight up **(dorsiflexion)** and down **(plantarflexion)**. The talus causes the foot to veer to the outside or inside depending on which direction you're moving. You'll notice it rotate slightly when pointing your foot up. If you then point you toes downward, you'll see that the sole of the foot now wants to point slightly to the inside. The shape of the talus helps make this happen.

So if the foot is on the ground and the knee is passing over it, the foot is moving into dorsiflexion, and the talus helps direct the lower leg and knee to the inside of the foot. This flattens the foot and the arch. The term given to describe this foot flattening is **pronation**.

Likewise, when the foot points downward into plantarflexion, the talus creates the opposite effect—that of moving the lower leg to the outside of the foot creating a higher arch. The term describing this higher arch position is **supination**. It gets more complicated than this, but that's as far as we'll go for now.

The Gait Cycle

The term **gait cycle** refers to how you walk. The gait cycle is com-prised of a stance phase and swing phase. The stance phase is when the foot is on the ground, and the swing phase is when the foot is swinging through the air to advance for the next step.

The stance phase has three parts: the heel strike (I like to say foot strike), where the foot has its initial contact with the ground; then the midstance, where the body is traveling over the foot; and fi-nally there is push-off (toe-off or heel-off), where the foot makes its final effort to advance the body forward. The end of the stance phase also prepares the foot and leg to swing through to accept the next step.

While all this is happening, there is an interplay of pelvic and shoulder rotation that helps maintain balance, forward motion, and proper muscle firing throughout the gait cycle. Essentially, the opposite arm and leg swings forward to create a counterbalanced forward movement. However, we rarely walk with our arms free, and so this sequence is often disrupted, which creates motor planning disturbances and consequent muscle imbalances. These imbalances are often at the root of our pain.

There is more variation to this, depending on who you talk to, but for our purposes, this is enough to understand the terms I'll use throughout the rest of this book.

> **Motor planning** refers to how we organize movement in our body. It is affected by how well we sense and therefore control our muscles as well as movement habits we have created throughout our life.

The most controversial parts of the gait cycle is how the foot should come into contact with the ground (foot strike) and how the foot should act as the body is passing over it (midstance). This is where I think we get into the most trouble, and this is what I initially target to help people with chronic foot and ankle pain.

Usually, during the stance phase, the heel strikes the ground, then the knee passes forward over the foot, and the foot pronates or flattens as we continue on in our walking pattern. The foot then begins to supinate or increase its arch again as we push off. The timing of this as well as the degree of arch flattening and raising is what causes foot pain, whether it is **plantar fasciitis**, **heel spurs**, **hammertoes**, **Morton's neuromas**, and even **bunions**. We'll talk about all these problems in more detail later.

The Muscles of the Foot and Lower Leg

Let's move on to the muscles that control all these bones and motions. Many of the muscles that directly control the foot begin in the lower leg, and a couple even begin in the upper leg, so we'll begin there and work our way down.

I'm going to break these muscles down into two groups: those that dorsiflex the foot and ankle (make the toes and foot point up) and those that plantarflex the foot and ankle (make the toes and foot point down). At this stage of the game, I'm just giving you the big picture of these muscles' functions. Please don't feel you need to memorize where they begin and end.

The Dorsiflexors

Four dorsiflexor muscles begin in the lower leg and insert onto the foot in some fashion or another to help point the toes upward (Figure 2.2).

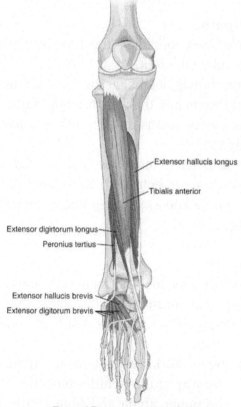

Extensor hallucis longus

Tibialis anterior

Extensor digirtorum longus

Peronius tertius

Extensor hallucis brevis

Extensor digitorum brevis

Dorsiflexors and Helpers

Figure 2.2 There are several muscles that help dorsiflex the foot and ankle.

The extensor digitorum longus begins on the outer part of the tibia, interosseous membrane, and fibula, and it inserts onto the tops of the four outer toes.

Peronius tertius begins on the lower part of the fibula and interosseous membrane, and it inserts onto the base of the fifth toe.

Extensor hallucis longus begins at the middle part of the fibula and interosseous membrane, and it inserts onto the base of the big toe.

Tibialis anterior begins on the outer portion of the tibia and interosseous membrane, and it inserts onto the inner part and underneath the first cuneiform bone (see Figure 2.1. for the locations of the bones)

Dorsiflexor Helpers

Two other muscles help dorsiflex the foot by lifting the toes. These begin and end on the foot.

Extensor digitorum brevis begins on the top and outer portion of the heel bone and inserts into the first through fourth toes.

Extensor hallucis brevis begins in the same area and inserts into the base of the big toe.

That's it. Just six muscles to move the foot into dorsiflexion! You use them when you walk to help keep your toes from scraping on the ground and tripping you as your leg moves forward during the swing phase of gait.

The Plantarflexors

Eight muscles plantarflex the foot and begin at the lower leg or above: The gastrocnemius (calf muscle) begins above the knee joint at the ends of the femur and inserts onto the heel bone (calcaneus) via the Achilles tendon.

Plantaris begins above the knee joint on the femur and inserts onto the heel bone by way of the Achilles tendon.

Soleus begins at the upper fibula and tibia and inserts, together with the calf muscle, onto the heel bone, again through the Achilles tendon.

Tibialis posterior begins on the fibula, tibia, and interosseous membrane and inserts onto the bottom of the navicular bone as well as all three cuneiforms.

Peroneous longus begins on the outer tibia and fibula and runs under the foot to insert onto the first metatarsal bone and first cuneiform.

Peroneus brevis begins on the lower fibula and inserts onto the 5th metatarsal bone.

Flexor hallucis longus begins at the mid fibula and interosseous membrane and runs under the foot to insert onto the base of the big toe.

Flexor digitorum longus begins at the mid tibia and runs under the foot to insert onto the base of the second through fifth toes.

If you look closely at the calf and soleus muscles' architecture, you'll notice they are broad and large and insert via the thick Achilles tendon into the heel bone—much different than the other muscles of the lower leg. The calf and soleus muscles are designed for heavy lifting, whereas I tend to see the other plantarflexors more as fine-tuning muscles, much like guy wires. They help the foot stay relatively stable, controlling pronation and supination, as they assist plantarflexion. Many of these plantarflexors attach to the bottom of the foot, helping to curl the toes downward or in some way control the arch of the foot.

Plantarflexor Helpers and Arch Supporters

Eight muscles curl the toes downward. I call them plantarflexor helpers because they in some ways support the function of the other plantarflexor muscles coming from the lower leg. They also support the arch and seem to be more easily activated during plantarflexion. Notice that they generally run lengthwise on the bottom of the foot. Aside from their individual actions, this group of muscles also helps combat excessive flattening of the arch (Figure 2.3).

Abductor hallucis begins at the inner heel bone and inserts onto the outer base of the big toe.

Adductor hallucis is a little complicated, but it essentially begins at the bases of the second, third, fourth, and fifth metatarsal heads and inserts into the outer base of the big toe.

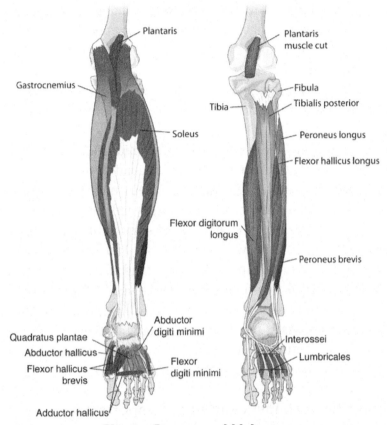

Plantarflexors and Helpers

Figure 2.3 The muscles on the bottom of the foot help with plantarflexion.

Flexor hallucis brevis begins on the undersurface of the cuboid and cuneiform bones and inserts onto the base of the big toe.

Flexor digitorum brevis begins on the inner half of the underside of the heel bone and inserts into the second through fifth toes.

Quadratus plantae begins on the underside of the heel bone and inserts onto the flexor digitorum longus.

Flexor digiti minimi begins at the base of the fifth metatarsal bone and inserts onto the fifth toe.

Lumbricales and interossei are little muscles that run in between the toes and assist with flexing the toes and may assist with extending them too depending on the position of the toes.

All these muscles cause the toes to grip, which also causes the arch to increase. You can test this yourself by curling the toes (all five of them!) downward into the ground. You will feel the arch rise up and the foot roll slightly outward as you do so.

One last idea to keep in mind is that although all these muscles appear to have a finite beginning and end, they actually don't. Fascia links all these muscles together. Remember, fascia is connective tissue that can be thick, as in the plantar fascia, or exist as thin weblike structures. It wraps around bundles of muscles, attaching to bone, ligaments, tendons, nerves, blood vessels, and other fascia. It is also innervated and can sense pressure and stretch. Lines of fascia travel throughout the body connecting our toes to our nose, leapfrogging across the musculoskeletal system. These fascial lines may cause changes in muscle function through developing a systemic tension that acts on our tissues.

The Five Biggest Contributors to Foot Pain

Believe it or not, there is a purpose to showing you all those bones and muscles. Even though I'm not asking you to memorize them, it's good to have a general idea of where they are and how they function (in terms of plantarflexion or dorsiflexion). In this section, we'll put a lot of this information together to help you understand why you may be having chronic foot pain.

Essentially foot pain (as well as other pain in the body) arises from stress created at whatever tissues are hurting. Regarding the foot, these stressors include foot strike or walking patterns, calf and soleus tightness, the shape of the foot in terms of pronation or supination, the shape of the thigh bones, and foot muscle dysfunction. All of these issues can come together creating chronic stress and pain to the foot and ankle system.

Keep in mind these are only the musculoskeletal reasons behind your pain. The underlying control of all these issues lies in your brain and your nervous and fascial systems, which we covered in the last chapter.

Walking Habits

I believe our human function follows our form. In other words, if our muscles indicate a certain function, then we should allow those muscles to perform that function to maintain harmony and decrease stress in that general anatomical area. If one muscle or a group of muscles aren't doing the job they were designed to do, excessive stress and tension is delivered to the area, if not to adjacent areas. This is especially true while walking, during which our body generates tremendous forces that need to be controlled while at the same time allowing it to remain relaxed and fluid.

Having said that, let's tally the results of our anatomy lesson. We have four foot and ankle dorsiflexors with two helpers amounting to six muscles controlling this motion. Then we have eight plantarflexors with six helpers (not counting the lumbricales or interossei because they sometimes go both ways), which gives us fourteen plantarflexors. Also two of those plantarflexors (the calf and soleus) have a unique design making them huge and powerful—the largest and strongest muscles in the lower leg by far.

Here's where I'm going with all this: if we have six muscles that help us dorsiflex the foot and we have fourteen muscles that control plantarflexion (two of which are the largest in the lower leg), then *why do we walk primarily using dorsiflexion and only let our plantarflexors come into the picture after our foot strikes the ground and we are traveling over it?*

Most people walk by reaching the leg out in front of them and striking the heel down on the ground, then advancing the hips and body over the foot. When the heel hits the ground the foot is in dorsiflexion, which means those muscles are working. The plantarflexors aren't working (Figure 2.4). Therefore we have tremendous ground reaction forces coming up through the foot at foot strike but 14 of our muscles (the plantarflexors) aren't being used to dampen this potential stress.

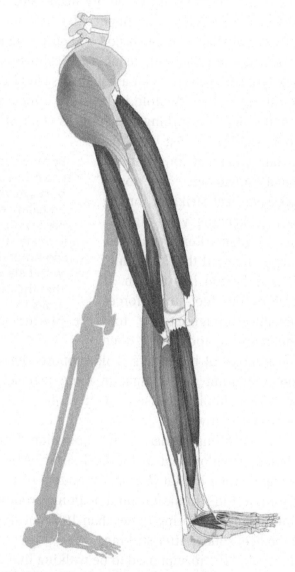

Walking Mechanics with Dorsiflexion
Figure 2.4 When heel striking while walking, emphasis is placed on the dorsiflexors and hamstrings.

WABASH CARNEGIE PUBLIC LIBRARY

Let's say you weigh 150 pounds and I am your foot. If you're about to fall on me from above and I have no choice but to catch you, then I want to put myself in the most mechanically advantaged position I can. It won't be on my heels because I don't get to use 14 of my muscles upon impact. I will want to use every muscle I have available to catch you and stay balanced. For that same person walking one mile using a typical heel-strike pattern, the shock absorption forces can amount to several tons, and running can increase them twofold.[1] Therefore it makes sense to recruit as many shock-absorbing structures as you can.

Your foot and lower leg need to accept your weight with as much mechanical advantage as possible. Excessive heel striking, for the most part, is keeping your big hitters, the 14 plantarflexor muscles, out of the game until the 7th inning, when it may be too late to win. If we distribute the foot-strike forces more evenly throughout the foot and sooner during foot strike, then we can use those 14 big hitters. This supports the arch and controls foot pronation and supination more precisely and earlier when walking. This is because, as you've just seen, many of the muscles from the lower leg insert onto the bottom of the foot to assist with controlling pronation and supination. I'm not advocating complete abandonment of the heel strike. After all, the heel bone is huge with a big fat pad on the bottom of it. It's supposed to bear weight. I just think it should be doing around 50% to 70% of the initial weight bearing rather than 100% of it. Or we should roll off the heel sooner after striking.

> Because your brain can sense more about your foot position with shoes off, and balance problems are often rooted in poor foot and ankle strategies, I often recommend to my clients with balance problems that they **walk without shoes** to improve neural connections to their brains.

You might ask, "If I'm supposed to be walking like that, then why aren't I?" Good question. The primary culprit is your shoes. Most shoes have a very thick heel—especially running or tennis shoes.

This thick heel essentially extends the length of the leg, allowing you to swing your leg out further in front of your body before striking your heel down. An interesting study was done with children that shows this.[2] A thick shoe heel also absorbs much of the trauma that would occur to your heel if you walked like this without the shoes on. Because the thick heels prevent you from feeling this trauma, you don't sense a need to change your walking pattern.

When I teach people to walk correctly, I always have them start in their bare feet, so they can feel the ground and what their feet are doing. Sensing the ground with your feet while standing and walking is foreign to most people (remember how important it is for your brain to be involved?). Once they master the techniques (presented in the following text), I ask them to put their shoes on and try it again. Most have a difficult time reproducing the correct walk in their shoes because the thick soles buffer the foot to the point where there is little or no feedback to the brain. I'm not advocating going around barefoot (although much of the world does). I'm talking about putting less shoe between you and the ground (especially at the heel) and slightly altering your foot-strike pattern so you can feel what you're doing and therefore resume control of your foot and ankle muscles.

How to Walk with Less Heel Strike

Learning to walk differently will be difficult because you've created deep neural pathways in your brain around this activity. You will have to become an outside observer of your own walking pattern to change it completely (remember the last chapter?). Initially, you will walk a little slower and it will take more effort. So there are short-term drawbacks to changing your behavior. You must keep your eye on the positive long-term benefits, however, such as a more energy-efficient walking pattern, little to no pain, and better muscle recruitment patterns resulting in less cumulative stress to your body.

To walk with less of a heel strike you'll initially have to take shorter steps—maybe 50% shorter. Doing so will allow your body to catch up to your advancing foot. Basically, your steps should be short enough so that, as the heel and/or midfoot strike the ground, your hips, pelvis, and trunk are lined up directly over your foot. They should be relaxed too.

This will be difficult for many of you because you're used to allowing your body to hang back while your foot advances. So take it slow and watch yourself in a mirror if possible to see that everything is stacked up at foot strike. I recommend practicing this with your shoes off so you can feel your foot interacting with the ground. You'll be able to feel that instead of just your heel striking the ground, your midfoot almost immediately comes into contact with the ground when your heel touches down. This will feel unnatural to you, but remember, that it doesn't mean it's bad. It's just different. You should feel your foot or calf muscles turning on sooner than usual during the stance phase of walking. One of the most common comments I hear is that my clients feel they are falling forward onto the advancing foot. That's exactly how you might feel when practicing this new technique.

That's it! As you get better, you'll be able to lengthen your stride again. In fact, your new walking pattern should look almost identical to your previous pattern but with the subtle difference that your body is lined up over your foot more at foot strike (Figure 2.5). This allows your foot, lower leg, and pelvic muscles to turn on sooner, controlling the foot and ankle better. The more you practice, the easier it will become to correct your gait pattern. I highly recommend setting aside two minutes 5 to 10 times a day to practice your new technique as well as frequent 30-second mental visualization periods during the first week to change your neural programming.[3] Once you've gotten this down, it will actually feel wrong to walk your old way.

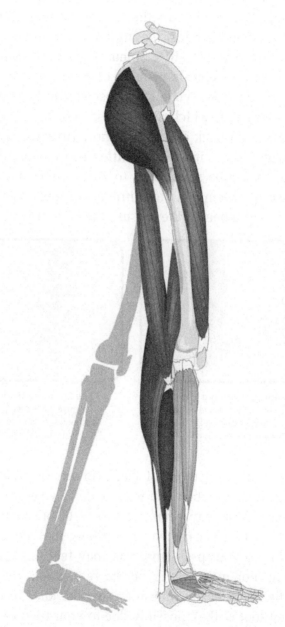

Walking Mechanics with Less Heel Strike

Figure 2.5 Walking with the pelvis over the foot at foot strike
helps turn on powerful plantarflexor muscles sooner.

Many of you will say, "But I already walk on my toes. What should I do?" First, check whether you are weight bearing through all five toes rather than just the big toe as in Figures 2.6 and 2.7. As you'll learn in the "Calf & Soleus Tightness" section, walking on the toes can present its own set of problems. By walking (or running) on your toes, your calf muscles can become shortened or more contracted, which also stresses the foot and ankle. The key, then, is to sit back on the foot more (using all five toes) and allow the heel to get involved a little bit. Remember, I think the heel strike should be about 50% to 70% of the initial strike: too much causes problems, but too little also causes problems. Learn to have more of a heel strike and use the arch of your foot more.

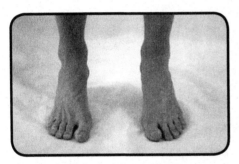 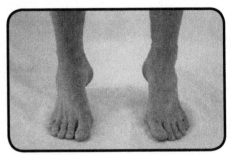

Toe Standing Using Big Toe
Figure 2.6 Many people who stand or walk on their toes do so with excessive weight bearing primarily on their big toe.

Toe Standing Using All Five Toes
Figure 2.7 Standing on all five toes distributes pressure to more muscles and areas of the plantar fascia.

As an experiment for those of you who are toe walkers, sit back on your heels more when you walk and see whether this decreases your pain. You may even need to walk on your heels to get the feel of it. If it does, then toe walking may be a habit that is contributing to your problems. You may feel this creates tension somewhere. For most it will be the realization your ankle does not dorsiflex very easily (doesn't allow the knee to pass over the foot during foot strike), possibly due to your tight calf muscles or ligament changes at the ankle joint. So transition slowly. There is a lot of force acting on your tissues—at least your body weight—so take it slow.

Becoming aware of how your walking pattern is contributing to your pain is a big part of fixing it. Usually it is because key muscles that control your joints or your arch are not activated soon enough (or are activated too much, in the case of toe walkers) in the gait cycle. When they do finally turn on, it is often too late to prevent damage.

The Shape of the Femur

Not everyone's thigh bones (femurs) are built the same. Some people's thigh bones are more twisted than others. If you've ever watched toddlers run, you'll notice their feet point inward. They are born with their femurs twisted inward, which is known as **anteversion**. As they grow, their femurs gradually twist outward to a normal alignment. On the other hand, some people's thigh bones twist out further than others. This is known as **retroversion**. These are just fancy words that mean the femur is either twisted inward more than normal (anteversion) or outward more than normal (Figures 2.8, 2.9, 2.10).

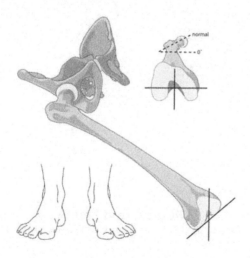

Normal Femur
Figure 2.8 A normal femur has some inward rotation of the shaft.

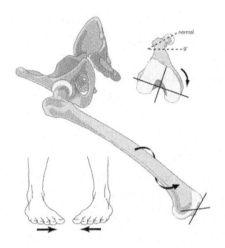

Anteverted Femur
Figure 2.9 Some people have a femur which is excessively twisted inward.

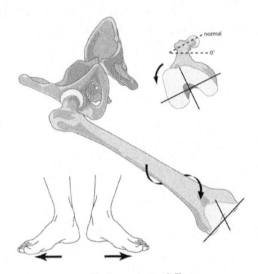

Retroverted Femur
Figure 2.10 Some people have a femur which is excessively twisted outward.

This in itself isn't a problem. The problem is that we all have an idea of how our feet should be pointed when we stand and walk—which is forward. But if our thigh bones are twisted, then this will change how our feet should be pointed. If we're not aware of this, then by pointing the feet forward, we are creating stress, often played out at the back, hip, knee, foot, and ankle—wherever you're most vulnerable.

An easy way to determine whether you have one or both femurs in anteversion or retroversion is to lie down on your stomach with both knees bent to 90 degrees and drop your feet to the outside. Then drop your feet to the inside. If you can drop your feet to the outside but not to the inside, as in the figures below (Figures 2.11a, b, & c), then you likely have anteverted femurs and your thigh bones are rotated inward (internally rotated).

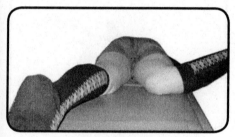

Anteverted Femur
Figure 2.11a This woman's right leg shows excessive internal rotation of the femur.

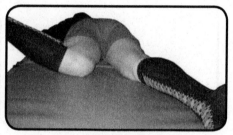

Anteverted Femur
Figure 2.11b This woman's left leg also shows excessive internal rotation of the femur.

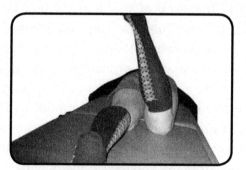

Anteverted Femur
Figure 2.11c This woman's right leg shows very little external rotation of the femur.

An anteverted femur is predisposed to excessive internal rotation, meaning the knees will point inward. In general, if you have anteverted femurs, then you need to have strong gluteal muscles to control this inward rotation. This is because the more the femur is allowed to rotate inward, the more the foot is driven into pronation, which stresses the foot tissues and joints. Strengthening your gluteal muscles, and using them when walking, will help control this excessive internal rotation and consequently foot pronation because they are external rotators of the thigh bone and, by extension, will help supinate the foot more (or at least reduce the forces contributing to pronation.

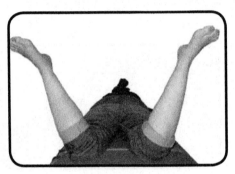

Retroverted Femur
Figure 2.12a This woman's legs show very little internal rotation of the femur.

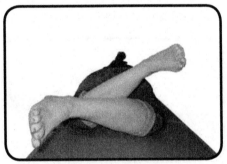

Retroverted Femur
Figure 2.12b This woman's legs show excessive external rotation of the femur.

The exercises in the back of this book, Glute Pumps, Standing Hip Tubes, and Lateral Tube Walking, all achieve this as well as learning how to walk better. Walking with less heel strike will keep the foot out of excessive pronation longer because the plantarflexor muscles are activated sooner in the gait cycle.

If, on the other hand, you have a lot of mobility dropping the feet to the inside but not the outside as in the figures above (Figures 2.12a & b), then you likely have retroverted femurs. This means your femurs are externally rotated (to the outside).

In this situation, you may be better off pointing your feet slightly outward. This is because by pointing the feet straight ahead, you are using up most of your available hip range of motion. Continuing to point the feet forward means you must increase your effort to control the gait cycle. This effort can be expressed in several ways such as pulling up the toes harder—which can contribute to hammertoes. Or the force of your femurs attempting to rotate back outward can potentially lead to Tailor's bunions, Morton's neuromas, chronic ankle sprains, or other issues.

If you have retroverted femurs, experiment with turning the knees and feet out a few degrees and see whether your foot and leg seem more relaxed in this position. Try to stay away from judging whether it feels "natural." It won't. You've already decided "natural" means pointing your feet forward. So just go by the level of stress you feel at work on your legs and feet.

It sometimes happens that one leg is more retro- or anteverted than another. In fact, I've seen people with one retroverted femur and one anteverted femur (which means they had some adjusting to do with their standing/walking habits!). So pay attention to your test and don't assume that one side of your body is the mirror image of the other.

The position of the shin bone (tibia) can also contribute to foot pain. Below is an image of a woman with anteverted femurs (Figure 2.13 a & b). You can see her knees are pointed inward but her feet are facing straight ahead. She not only had foot pain

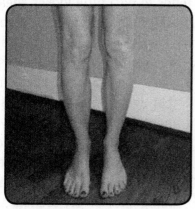

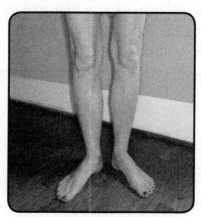

Anteverted Femurs Standing
Figure 2.13a Note this woman's knees point inward but the feet are straight.

Anteverted Femurs
Corrected Standing
Figure 2.13b Pointing the knees forward reduced her pain.

but also knee, hip, and back pain. She was a dancer. When someone has pain all through the lower extremities, I first try to correct where the knee and hip needs to be to unload stress above and below these joints. When we turned her knees out slightly (Figure 2.13b) so they were facing forward (instead of pointing in), she instantly felt less stress and pain throughout her lower extremities. She didn't like the fact that her feet pointed out so much. That is an aesthetic value, however, and shouldn't take precedence over painful movement habits.

Her lower leg outward rotation is due to an alignment issue that the tibia developed, I believe, as a consequence of her extensive ballet training. Because of this excessive tibial rotation, she had to turn her thighs in to make it appear the feet were pointing forward. This excessive effort created pain throughout her legs and back.

Shape and Mobility of the Foot & Ankle

It doesn't take a genius to see that everyone's feet are shaped differently. There are high arches, low arches, wide feet, narrow feet, long feet, and short feet—and all sorts of combinations of these general shapes. We'll just be focusing on high and low arches.

A flatter foot (one with low arches) is said to be pronated (Figure 2.14). In general, a pronated foot tends to be a little looser, meaning the ligaments and muscles are slightly sluggish in their jobs of controlling the joints. This makes sense because the fact that the arch is sitting lower usually means the structures that would hold it up (ligaments and muscles), must be longer, weaker, or both. Most people's feet have a tendency toward flatness rather than being excessively arched.

So if the tissues are longer or weaker, they generally will

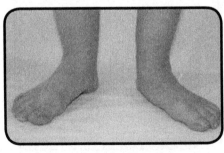

Pronated Feet
Figure 2.14. Note the arches of these feet nearly touch the ground. Her left foot is more pronated than her right.

undergo more stress when asked to work because they are unused to generating ample tension to control the foot. This is especially important for ligament integrity because the ligaments are the primary stabilizers of joints. Muscles are secondary stabilizers. If lax ligaments aren't controlling the foot well and the load falls to muscles, then stress develops, as well as risk of injury.

A rigid, higher-arched, or supinated foot can cause problems too (Figure 2.15). I don't see many feet with this profile, but they do exist and have problems associated with their rigidity. The tissues on the bottom of these feet are often too short or contracted—the opposite of the pronated foot's issues.

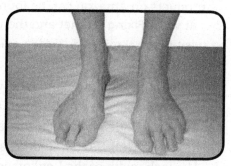

Supinated Feet

Figure 2.15. The arches of these feet rest high off the ground. Her right foot is more supinated than her left.

If you're interested in how your foot shape stacks up, go outside in your bare feet and walk through a puddle on the concrete to see what your imprint looks like. Here is a general guide of how different foot shapes appear (Figure 2.16).

Okay, so let's say you've just discovered you have a pronated or supinated foot. How can you change its shape? It's not so much that you change the shape of your foot; the forces acting on the shape are what matter. The shape of your foot gives you clues as to what the tissues (which are painful) must be going through. The goal is to unload tissue stress. I use a very simple taping process to unload the foot to see how that effects pain. Usually just one strip will do it (actually two strips, one on top of the other). But you

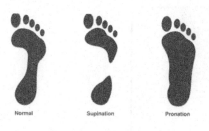

Normal   Supination   Pronation

Foot Imprints

Figure 2.16 Looking at the imprint of a foot can give information as to the weight bearing patterns and shape.

Cover Roll Stretch and **Leukotape P** can be purchased on **Amazon** or several other websites. Typical athletic tape purchased in stores will stretch out too quickly and therefore be ineffective. Links to these products on Amazon can be found at **www.FixingYou.net** and then visiting on the Foot & Ankle page.

need the right tape. It must be strong to hold up against all those weight-bearing forces and able to stay on even after bathing.

I use two types of tape. The first is called CoverRoll Stretch. I use the 2-inch width. This is laid down first and protects your skin from the second tape, Leukotape P, which is a very strong tape. It also has a tendency to break down the skin and cause blisters or even tear off a little skin when the tape is removed. That's why we use the CoverRoll Stretch underneath it—to protect the skin. I use the 1½-inch width of the Leukotape P.

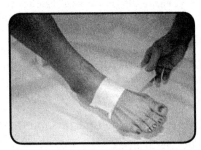

Taping a Pronated Foot
Figure 2.17a Taping to control foot pronation.

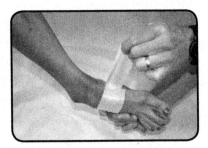

Taping a Pronated Foot
Figure 2.17b Pulling up on the tape, lifts the arch.

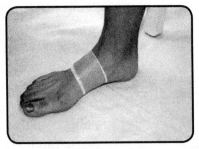

Taping a Pronated Foot
Figure 2.17c Standing with a correctly taped foot should feel less painful.

Also, because of this skin breakdown issue, I often recommend wearing it for 1 or 2 hours and no more than half a day the first time out (even less if you have fair or sensitive skin) just to make sure your skin can handle it. Especially if you have sensitive skin or thin skin from medications, please consult your physician prior to applying this tape.

Figures 2.17 a, b, & c show my taping technique which can also be found as videos on my website, www.FixingYou.net. Essentially, with a flatter foot, I will tape to pull the arch up dramatically. This unloads the tissues supporting the arch, including the muscles, ligaments, and **plantar fascia**. As with all new treatments, please consult your physician, who is familiar with your particular issues, before taping or attempting any new exercise.

One easy test to help determine if you are loose-jointed is to straighten your arms out in front of you. If your elbows bend backwards a little, then you are more than likely loose jointed. This can be confirmed if you can easily bend your knees slightly backward knees and/or fingers backward too.

With a higher, rigid foot I will tape to bring the arch down (Figure 2.18). The goal here is to give the foot more mobility and bring it out of its rigid pattern. We are trying to lengthen the tissues on the bottom, teaching the foot and ankle to relax more, rather than allowing them to remain in a shortened position and relatively unused.

It's important to understand that you could have one pronated foot and one supinated foot, just as you can have one retroverted femur and one anteverted femur. In fact, this is not uncommon. So you may use two completely different taping strategies for your feet.

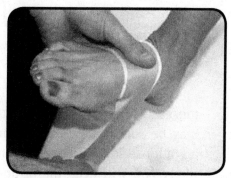

Taping a Supinated Foot
Figure 2.18 Taping a supinated foot involved gently pulling the arch out of its rigid position.

I'd like to point out that you will feel you are walking different-ly with this tape on your feet. Pay attention to these changes (es-pecially if your pain decreases) because the tape is teaching you how to walk better. But ultimately you must control your walk-ing pattern. The tape will never trump your intrinsic movement habits; it will only disrupt them temporarily.

Matching your walking pattern to correct your foot structure is a powerful tool to equalize pressures acting through your feet. Again, it will feel completely foreign, but that's the point. We want to change how you're doing things because your current habits are causing you pain. The tape is helping you understand what those changes should be.

Loose Ankles

But all the blame doesn't just fall on the foot; it falls on the ankle joint too. Remember all those ligaments holding the ankle togeth-er back in Figure 2.1 (page 28). There's a reason for those. We need stability! Often there is excessive laxity of the ankle ligaments, es-pecially in people with chronic ankle pain or recurrent sprains.

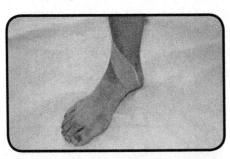

Taping for Loose Ankles
Figure 2.19 Supporting the ankle with tape is often helpful in controlling foot pronation.

My taping technique for the ankle also uses just one piece of tape (Figure 2.19). although it's a little trickier to do. Quite often the breakdown of the ankle is the culprit causing pain, in which case foot orthoses may be appro-priate, depending on the severity of the problem (see "Foot Or-thoses" on page 74). You'll know more about how your ankles may be contributing to your problem after they are taped. If you are a loose-jointed person with very loose ankles, then it is more likely you will need the orthoses. This is because, in my experi-ence, loose ankles are just tougher to overcome with training.

The taping technique shown in Figure 2.19 is for a foot and ankle that is excessively flat and collapses inward. The spiraling tape helps supports the foot and ankle and pulls it out of this stressful position. Other ankle taping techniques are mentioned later in the "Ankle Sprain" section beginning on page 72. Again, please consult with your physician, who is familiar with your condition, prior to taping your ankles or feet.

Callus Pattern

In addition to making a foot imprint on paper, another clue to weight-bearing patterns is to look at the calluses on the bottoms of your feet. Callus forms from repeated rubbing of the skin (Figure 2.20a, b & c). If a foot pronates, you will often see a callus formed on the part of the big toe that is more toward your

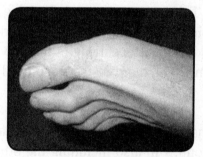
Callus Pattern
Figure 2.20a No callus pattern is noted on this big toe.

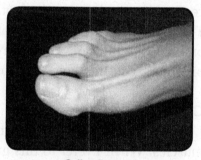
Callus Pattern
Figure 2.20b An inner toe callus pattern is noted on this big toe.

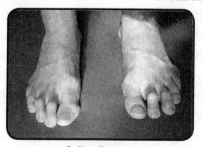
Callus Pattern
Figure 2.20c Comparing callus patterns between feet gives clues as to weight bearing tendencies.

midline. It's very common to find this callus formed on one toe but not another. This is an indication that one foot is more pronated than the other and can help you understand how you might tape your feet or adapt your walking pattern.

For instance, if you found the callus pattern on the inner big toe of the foot that is in pain, you might come to the conclusion that foot is pronating too much and would focus on taping that arch up. Also, when walking you might try changing your foot-strike pattern to decrease the heel strike, which activates the plantarflexors sooner and prevents it from fully collapsing in. Also pay attention to the other leg's role in this. Does it avoid bearing weight? Perhaps the painful foot is falling victim to the other leg's issues.

When only one foot has a big toe callus pattern, there is often a larger issue at work that begins at the pelvis (See, *Fixing You: Hip & Knee Pain*). Often I see a systemic breakdown that leads to excessive stress collapsing the foot. This happens in one or both legs.

The bigger picture in this scenario is that different callus patterns on each foot indicates there may be issues occurring in the pelvis or femurs, causing them to become rotated or twisted as you walk.

Calf & Soleus Tightness

Let's look at another system that can stress the foot—the calf muscles. When I refer to this group, I'm also including the other lower leg plantarflexors. It's difficult to have tightness in just one or two muscles so we'll just consider them all together but focus mainly on the calf and soleus muscles because they attach directly into the back of the heel from the lower leg, and even the femur.

As the knee passes over the foot, the calf muscles must lengthen enough to allow the ankle joint to bend. The stiffer this muscle group is, the more difficult it will be for the ankle joint to bend. The calf muscles should be absorbing some of the weight of the body by lengthening as the knee passes over the foot. Instead, by not lengthening, they are acting like a long lever against the foot's arch, because that is the next most mobile part of the foot and ankle complex (Figure 2.21). The arch then absorbs this excessive repeated stress by collapsing and transmits that stress to any number of tissues within the foot. On top of that, if the muscles haven't been prepared to support the arch (as when using a strong heel-strike walking pattern), they will be more vulnerable to injury. This is often a major contributor to plantar fasciitis and heel spurs.

The arch, in addition to being designed to collapse naturally, is composed of a lot of different bones, which means it can absorb force at a lot of different places. The excessive force from the stiff calf muscles can overload any one or several of those joints, stretching and stressing the soft tissues on the bottom of the foot, such as ligaments, nerves, and muscles, as the arch is driven downward. So we need to lengthen the calf muscles and allow the ankle joint to bend better to reduce this stress.

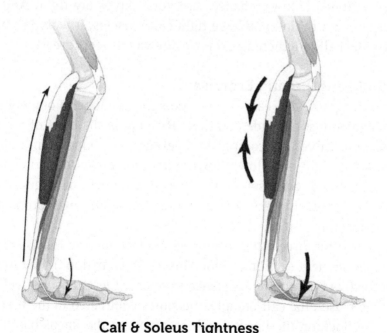

Calf & Soleus Tightness

Figure 2.21 The image on the left shows that when the calf muscles are lengthened, less force is transmitted to the arch because the knee can travel over the ankle and foot. The image on the right depicts excessive force through the arch due to calf tightness and the inability of the knee to travel over the foot and ankle.

I've found that traditional calf stretches sometimes work for some people, but are usually ineffective for those with chronic problems. One reason is because the brain has learned that the current state of contraction of those muscles is the one most used and therefore reinforced. Stretching these muscles will not teach the brain to lengthen them and, therefore, they will contract again.

Instead, I recommend the calf-lengthening exercise below together with changing your footstrike pattern. The key to this exercise is to sense the gently contracted calf muscles while they are lengthening in order to achieve a more permanent resting length and tension. This teaches the brain to allow them to lengthen.

How do you determine if you need to lengthen your calves? Good question. In my experience, I've learned to just ask my patients. Most people know whether their calves are tight or not. Also, if you stand or walk with hyperextended knees or walk on your toes (mentioned below), chances are your calves are tight. And even if you don't think you have tight calf muscles, it wouldn't hurt to try the calf lengthening exercise anyway. It feels great!

Calf Lengthening Exercise

To lengthen the calf muscle complex, stagger your stance to lengthen just one side at a time. Rise up on the balls of your foot so your calves are contracted. Feel the calf contraction. Lean forward slightly, and slowly lower your heel down to the floor while maintaining your sense of the calf contraction (Figures 2.22a & b). Gradually lessen that contraction as the heel drops down. Repeat three times.

I also offer three other lower-leg and foot muscle release exercises in the next section ("Foot Muscle Dysfunction") that are quite effective but require assistance to release these muscles well.

One reason the calf complex becomes contracted in the first place is by locking the knees (such as snapping the knees back) when standing or walking. This pushes the knee joint slightly behind the ankle joint. When this is habitual, the calf muscles shorten.

Unlocking your knees will feel unfamiliar to you, but this is necessary to train your body (and your brain) to use them in a lengthened position.

One highly effective method I use to help people discover how pervasive this is, and unlock their knees more frequently, is to tape the backs of their legs (Figure 2.23). While they stand with soft knees, I simply put tape along the back of their legs, crossing the knee joint. That way, when they try to straighten their knees, they will feel the tug of the tape (especially if they have hairy legs!). You'll be amazed at how often you do this when standing or walking!

Another reason the calf muscles become tight is due to habitu-

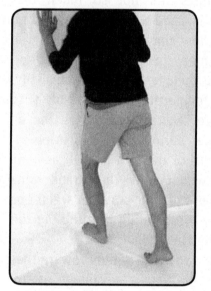 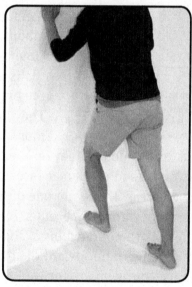

Calf Lengthening Exercise
Figure 2.22a Begin with the heel up in the air and calf muscle contracted.

Calf Lengthening Exercise
Figure 2.22b Finish by lowering the heel down, maintaining a gentle contraction in the calf muscles.

al toe walking. Some people walk or run on the balls of their feet. Their heels remain relatively unused. This teaches the brain to keep the calf and foot muscles contracted and shortened because they are rarely given the opportunity to lengthen when function-

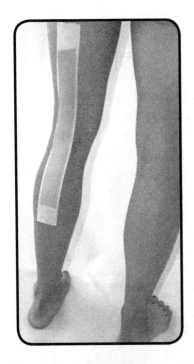

Taping for Knee Hyperextension
Figure 2.23 A strip of tape along the back of the leg when the knee is slightly bent will help eliminate knee hyperextension.

ing. Again, this leads to excessive stress to the foot because the arch is not permitted to lengthen, shorten, and bear weight as it was designed to do. So, when considering foot-strike patterns, toe walkers have gone a little too far in the opposite direction of heel striking. They need to involve the heel more by allowing it to strike, if only a little bit. This will dramatically change the dynamics of the foot and ankle, so do this gradually and slowly.

Sometimes it's not so much that a person is a toe walker but instead more about *how* they are toe walking. I've found many people run or walk on the balls of their feet almost exclusively on the big toe portion of the ball of the foot. They are practically ignoring the other four toes during weight bearing. This puts tremendous strain on the ball of the foot as well as along a narrow strand of plantar fascia, which makes that strand vulnerable to stress. If you are one of these people, consider weight bearing more through the outer four toes, rolling into the big toe as you walk (mentioned in "Walking Habits").

By striking more toward the outer foot and rolling toward the big toe as you advance forward, you will take advantage of stress-dampening elements of these outer tissues. Again, this will involve using foot and ankle muscles as well as their associated joints in a way they are not accustomed to being used, so make these changes gradually. Give yourself time to fine-tune the techniques to make them right for you. You will be changing deep neural pathways in your brain around this pattern, so go slowly. If it is right for you, you should feel rapid pain relief, even though the walking pattern will feel completely unnatural. Go by your pain response rather than whether it feels different or not.

Finally, one more habit that contributes to calf tightness is sleep. Most people sleep with their ankles in plantarflexion because the blankets or sheets may be pulling them in this direction. Or perhaps that's just the way they've decided to sleep. Regardless, that means the plantarflexor muscles are kept in a shortened position for 6 to 9 hours each night. That's a lot of time spent in this position, and it may be undoing all the lengthening you are achieving throughout the day, making you start from square one in the morning again. Wearing night splints is a simple solution to this problem.

Night splints are designed to keep the plantarflexor muscles lengthened. Many of you reading this may have tried night splints already and not received much benefit. But when you look at foot and ankle pain as a result of several possible factors, then you may want to think twice about discontinuing them if you have tight calves. It may be that you need to address the other factors contributing to your pain, in addition to your tight calves, to remedy your situation. So give them another try while you also address the other issues discussed in this book.

There are two common types of night splints: the boot and the dorsal night splint (Figure 2.24 and 2.25). As you might imagine there are pros and cons to both. The boot is usually adjustable, so you can set the desired amount of tension on your calf complex. The problem with the boot is that it's bulky, and many people have a hard time sleeping with it on.

The dorsal night splint takes care of this problem by being lightweight and comfortable. The problem with the dorsal night splint is that they usually are not adjustable, so you may not get the lengthening you need. However, keep in mind that we are merely trying to prevent the calf muscles from shortening while you sleep, rather than trying to stretch them, so the dorsal night splint may be adequate for this purpose.

Foot Muscle Dysfunction

If you remember from the beginning of our anatomy lesson, the bottom of the foot has quite a few muscles in it including the

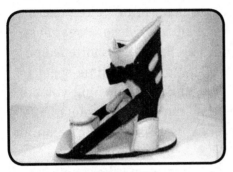

Boot Night Splint
Figure 2.24 A boot night splint allows adjustments in tension but is more bulky than dorsal night splints.

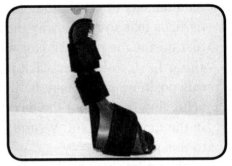

Dorsal Night Splint
Figure 2.25 Dorsal night splints are generally lighter weight and less bulky than boot splints.

flexor digitorum brevis muscle, which mirrors the plantar fascia (Figure 2.26). Also, many of the lower leg muscles insert onto the bottom of the foot, which makes it a very busy territory. Many of these muscles have been functionally silent (but irritated!) due to some of the stressors acting on them we've already mentioned. Consequently, they will need to be trained to unload the overloaded and strained tissues. Just beginning to walk again using a different foot-strike pattern will help, but many of you will need a more concentrated effort to get these muscles working well again and restore their normal resting length and tension.

Here are a few simple but powerful exercises to reeducate these muscles and reacquaint them with your brain. The first two exercises, Plantarflexor Muscle Lengthening Parts 1 and 2, address the plantarflexors of the lower leg. The third, Foot Muscle Lengthening, targets smaller individual muscles on the bottom of the foot as well as the calf and soleus muscles. It will be best if someone helps you with these exercises.

Flexor digitorum longus and plantar fascia

Figure 2.26 The flexor digitorum longus
mirrors the plantar fascia.

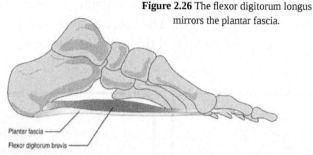

Plantar fascia ———

Flexor digitorum brevis ———

Before doing them, stand up (in your bare feet) and assess how your feet feel. Assess how high the arch is on the floor and how your toes rest on the floor. Also note any tension in your ankles, calves, or hips. Perform the exercises on one foot and then stand up to note the differences between the two feet. Then perform them on the other foot.

Plantarflexor Muscle Lengthening

This exercise is complicated to describe in words and so I will ask you to visit the website (www.FixingYou.net) to watch the video. I'll describe the exercise here in general terms. Always be sure to consult your physician, who is familiar with your particular issues, prior to performing these exercises.

Part 1

Lie down on your back and bring your foot and ankle into plantarflexion and eversion (scoop the foot downward and outward). This contracts the outer calf muscles, putting them in a shortened position. Your helper tries to move the forefoot inward and applies only enough resistance to the foot to help you sense the muscles that are contracting (Figure 2.27a & b). Your partner slowly first rolls the foot in (scooping inward) while you gently resist that motion, so you can feel those muscles contracting while they are lengthening. Once the foot is rolled inward, while maintaining their resistance, allow your foot to move into dorsiflexion to further lengthen the muscles while you are gently contracting them. This is not a battle of strength. The resistance should be only as much as necessary for you to feel the muscles, no more. Repeat 3 times.

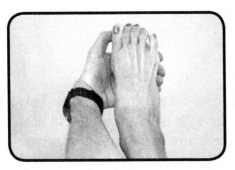 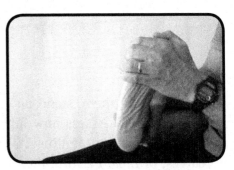

Plantarflexor Muscle Lengthening Part 1
Figure 2.27a Begin with the foot pointing outward. Apply gentle pressure pulling it inward and then into dorsiflexion.

Plantarflexor Muscle Lengthening Part 1
Figure 2.27b Allow your foot to move inward and up (into dorsiflexion) very slowly. Your partner continues to apply gentle pressure throughout the full range of motion.

Part 2

The second part releases the muscles on the inside of the lower leg and calf. You will bring your foot and ankle into plantarflexion and inversion (scoop the foot inward and downward). This contracts the inner calf muscles, putting them in a shortened position (Figure 2.28a & b). Your helper pulls the forefoot outward, applying only enough resistance to the foot to help you sense the muscles that are contracting. Your partner slowly first rolls the foot out (scooping outward) while you gently resist that motion, so you can feel those muscles contracting while they are lengthening. Once the foot is rolled outward, while maintaining their resistance, allow your foot to move into dorsiflexion to further lengthen the muscles while you are contracting them. Again, this is not a battle of strength. The resistance should be only as much as necessary for you to feel the muscles, no more. Repeat 3 times

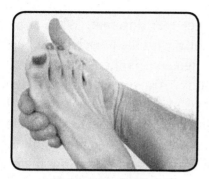

**Plantarflexor Muscle
Lengthening Part 2**

Figure 2.28a Begin with the foot pointing inward. Apply gentle pressure pulling it outward and then into dorsiflexion.

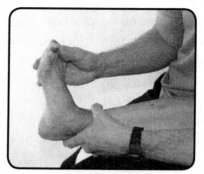

**Plantarflexor Muscle
Lengthening Part 2**

Figure 2.28b Allow your foot to move outward and up (into dorsiflexion) very slowly. Your partner continues to apply gentle pressure throughout the full range of motion.

Foot Muscle Lengthening

Your helper will put his or her fingers on the bottoms of your toes as well as on the balls of the foot, gently resisting them while you curl your toes down to create a fist with your foot (Figure 2.29a & b). Your helper should try to gently resist each toe in the process. See if you can even make the arch curl. We want to engage all the muscles of the bottom of the foot. Be sure your back and pelvis remain relaxed. Now, allow your partner to smoothly unroll your foot and toes until it is completely lengthened again while you gently resist, sensing the contraction of the foot muscles. Gentle resistance must be maintained through the full range of motion and through all five toes. Repeat 3 times.

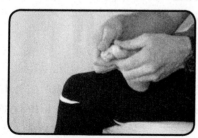

Foot Muscle Lengthening

Figure 2.29a Begin with fingers on each toe and the ball of the foot. Curl the foot down (plantarflexion) offering gentle resistance with the fingers.

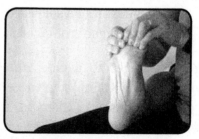

Foot Muscle Lengthening

Figure 2.29b Allow the foot to be brought slowly into dorsiflexion.

Stand up and assess how your feet feel different. Walk around and see how they function differently with the muscles in a better resting (and working) length and tension. Is there less pain? Do your feet rest on the floor differently? Are you walking differently? These last three exercises have introduced your brain to the muscles of the lower leg and foot. You've just established a new resting tension and length of those muscles. Your brain now has an improved ability to sense the muscles and can allow them to remain longer and more relaxed, yet perform just as well.

For many of you, this will eliminate your pain; however, it may return. If it does, you can repeat these exercises but you should realize that your pain is likely coming back because of how you are using your feet and lower legs. Take the time to experiment with your walking pattern to see if this is your culprit. Sense whether you hyperextend your knees backward, which causes excessively tight calf muscles. Find out whether your femurs are ante- or retroverted, and adjust your walking pattern accordingly or strengthen the appropriate muscles. All of the issues mentioned above have a role to play in your function and pain.

Okay, we've covered what I believe are the five biggest stressors causing foot and ankle pain:

1. Poor walking habits
2. The shape of the thigh bones
3. The shape and mobility of the foot and ankle
4. Chronic calf and soleus contraction
5. Poor awareness or control of the foot muscles

You will need to decide which are the biggest issues affecting your pain. The first step to getting better is being aware of what your problems are. Take your time to assess yourself and discover where it is you need help.

Common Foot & Ankle Problems

There are many different kinds of foot problems. I've listed a few of the most common ones below. The five mechanical issues I've just discussed are at the roots of most of them. Foot problems manifest differently in different people based on genetics, ligament laxity, history of use, traumas, or other variables.

When performing your exercises, be patient and take the time to sense and understand whether a particular exercise is actually helping or hurting. Documenting your pain level is a great way to track progress or lack thereof. If you see a trend of decreasing pain, then stick with whatever you are doing. You will get there. Try adding another exercise on top of that to see if it expedites your recovery. You must think about and sense what you're doing. If you see a trend of increasing pain, then try to tweak the exercises. If that still doesn't work, then take a moment to think about why your pain might be increasing. Use this as an opportunity to learn about your specific issues. Write down a hypothesis why your pain is increasing and what you should do to correct it, then test it to see if you're right. You must become your own therapist.

Plantar Fasciitis

The plantar fascia is a thick nonmuscular tissue that connects the heel bone to the base of the metatarsal heads. Remember, it also connects (indirectly) all the way up to your head (Figure 1.1, page 4), so issues along this fascial line may feed down to the foot.

The plantar fascia supports the arch of the foot. Plantar fasciitis is an inflammation of the plantar fascia. Like many medical diagnoses, this term only describes what is wrong with the tissue, not what is causing the inflammation.

The suffix **-itis** means inflammation. So plantar fasciitis is inflammation of the plantar fascia.

The classic symptom of plantar fasciitis is a tearing feeling on the bottom of the foot in the morning when you wake up and take your first steps. As the day progresses, the tearing feeling may go away and be replaced by a minor ache or no pain at all. In most people, the plantar fascia is irritated because it is overly stretched and therefore overly stressed. This is contrary to what most people believe is the problem—that the fascia is too tight. People with chronic plantar fasciitis may exhibit one or all five of the stressors mentioned above: poor walking habits, tight calf and soleus, flat feet, weak foot muscles, or rotated femurs. In most people I've worked with, just changing their walking patterns eliminates most of their pain because it activates the muscles of the foot earlier in the gait cycle, which reduces arch flattening and improves arch control.

However, I've worked with many more complicated cases where all five of these issues are present. If you are one of these people and typically lock your knees while standing, I highly encourage you to tape the backs of your knees or try the night splints. This will break the calf-tightening habits contributing to your pain.

Of course, if you have an overly stretched plantar fascia and you keep it stretched out at night, using a plantar fasciitis strap so it can't return to its proper length, you will not experience the painful tearing in the morning. But the longer-term consequences of this, especially for those who have flatter feet, is excessive lengthening of the plantar fascia, which is critical for arch support and overall foot function. Your arch would become even less stable as a consequence.

The foot taping technique I've described above (in the section titled, "Shape and Mobility of the Foot and Ankle") almost completely eliminates plantar fascia pain in the first few days the foot is taped. The tape is a temporary crutch to help remove the stress to the fascia, which allows it to heal while you are correcting the other issues that are driving the irritation.

Trigger-Point Release

Working out painful trigger points on the bottom of the foot can expedite recovery. You can do this by practicing the foot release

A **trigger point** is a bundle of knotted muscular or fascial tissue which, when pressed, can cause pain locally or in a more distant area of the body. Often, the presence of trigger points changes the muscle's function.

exercises above or using a golf ball (Figure 2.30). Simply place the golf ball under the foot on a point of tenderness and gradually increase pressure on it.

Maintain this pressure until the pain goes away and then move on to the next point, or put more pressure on the ball to more deeply release the trigger point. By releasing painful trigger points, you help to restore normal length and tension to the muscles, thereby improving their function. All this is nice if you're a heel striker, but what if you already forefoot strike (walk on your toes)? This can be a problem too. I've learned that forefoot strikers' calf muscles are usually too tight because their feet are kept in plantarflexion.

For these people, getting them to strike with more midfoot or heel strike is difficult because they don't have the calf length to allow it. You must correct this gradually.

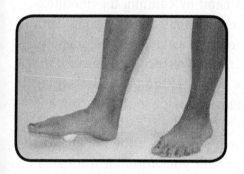

Golf Ball Release
Figure 2.30 Using a golf ball to work out painful trigger points can help restore motion to the foot muscles.

Heel Spurs

Heel spurs are painful bony growths where the plantar fascia meets the heel bone. The body often grows bone in areas of excessive stress; it's one of the ways it tries to protect itself. The heel spur may be formed due to excessive stress placed on that insertion point by the plantar fascia. Apparently, in some people, rather than the plantar fascia becoming overly stretched out, the stress is passed on to its insertion point on the heel. A bony growth ensues, creating a heel spur. Regardless, the same issues may be at play here.

While working on these issues, you can purchase a gel heel pad for your shoe in most pharmacies. I like to cut out a hole where the spur is to completely unload it. The less irritation to the spur, the greater chance for healing.

It goes without saying that you should employ all the treatments for plantar fasciitis to your heel spur problem. This includes changing your walk, taping the foot, lengthening the foot muscles, taping the back of your knees if you lock them out, and performing the neural correction exercises above.

Hammertoes

Hammertoe is a clawlike deformity where the knuckles of the toes bend upward, sometimes so much so that they rub against the top of the shoes and form unsightly calluses.

If you watch someone with hammertoes sit down and stand up, you'll notice the toes jump up every time they move. That happens because they've learned to overly recruit their dorsiflexors to walk, sit, and stand. Keeping the weight forward through the arch and toes will help reduce this habit by calming the dorsiflexors and recruiting the plantarflexors instead. This is a strong habit in people with this issue so it will require awareness and practice. Also when walking, the dorsiflexors are overrecruited because the pelvis is not over the foot at foot strike. If the pelvis is lagging behind the foot, then extra effort must be made to lift the foot and advance it. This extra effort comes from the dorsiflexors, which then pull up on the toes. If you heel strike, then the dorsiflexors must work harder and longer to prevent your forefoot from slapping down at foot strike.

Calf and soleus tightness contributes to this phenomena because they oppose the ankle dorsiflexors. If the calf and soleus are contracted, then the dorsiflexors must work harder to pull the foot up into dorsiflexion so the toes don't drag on the ground. Lengthening these muscles using the calf lengthening exercises will be beneficial.

Becoming aware of whether you have ante- or retroverted femurs and changing your foot-strike pattern accordingly can also help. If you have retroverted thigh bones, ones where the thigh bone is twisted outward slightly, yet you walk with your foot pointed forward, then you are working outside of your ideal range of motion. By turning your foot to face forward, you have used up much of your femur's internal rotation. This then requires more effort on your part to lift and advance your foot. Again, in people with hammertoes, this effort is driven by the ankle dorsiflexors, which insert into the toes. Releasing the foot muscles can also help restore normal foot muscle strength and function.

Morton's Neuromas

This is a benign neuroma located on a nerve that runs between the toes, usually the third and fourth toes. Some people don't believe it is a tumor at all but, instead, believe it is a fibrous tissue that surrounds the nerve. These may feel like you have a small pebble or marble between your toes. They can be quite painful. You could also experience burning or numbness as a result.
We must consider what is acting on that nerve that is causing the irritation. We should take into account all the information above to unravel the mystery. Our main goal will be to unload the stress being placed on that nerve. Once again, begin with calf and foot muscle lengthening as well as changing your foot-strike pattern for beginners.

Tailor's Bunions

Tailor's bunions are painful masses at the base of the pinky toe. I haven't seen many of these cases, but the few I've seen have involved the same issues mentioned earlier. Retroverted femurs seem to play a larger roll in these issues, however. In this case, the force of the femurs trying to rotate outward caused the foot to roll to the outside, increasing weight bearing on the pinky toe and forming the Tailor's bunion. Pain can almost immediately be reduced by rotating the feet and knees outward just a few degrees to match the rotation of the femur, although the bunion will take longer to disappear. Again, due to the stress of the rotated femurs, begin with calf and foot muscle lengthening as well as changing your foot-strike pattern.

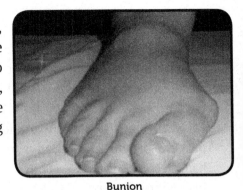

Bunion

Figure 2.31 A bunion has a characteristic bony prominence at the base of the big toe while the toe migrates inward.

Bunions

Bunions have a characteristic large bony bump at the base of the big toe due to one of the bones (the first metatarsal) migrating to the side (Figure 2.31). Often the toe itself migrates inward, accentuating the bony lump, sometimes to the point where it pushes the second toe upward and out of the way. The medical term is Hallux valgus. "Hallux" means big toe, and "valgus" refers to the outward migration of the bone.

These can become quite painful, not to mention unsightly. Surgery has been the only solution to correct these issues from an aesthetic standpoint. There are lots of splints on the market designed to help pull the toe back into place, but I've never heard that these splints actually correct the bunion.

I have had great success eliminating pain from bunions through correcting foot-strike patterns mentioned earlier. By using a midfoot strike, rather than a heel strike, the foot seems to remain in more of a supinated (higher-arched) position during the stance phase of gait. This supinated position theoretically draws the first metatarsal (the long bone that sticks out to the side in people with bunions) inward.[4]

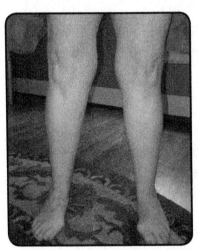

Ankle Collapse with Bunion

Figure 2.32 Bunions are often accompanied by ankles rolling inward.

I have to stress that this has only corrected pain associated with bunions, not the bunion formation itself. In many (but not all) of the feet I see with bunions, the ankle and foot arch seem to collapse (Figure 2.32). There seems to be excessive laxity in the ligaments holding the arch up, or excessive force driving into the foot. In figure 2.32, you can see this woman's knee rotates inward, driving down the arch of the foot. This is in conjunction with a hypermobile foot whose ligaments appear to be excessively stretched.

> When a joint moves too much relative to adjacent joints, it is susceptible to tissue breakdown and pain. The joint is said to be hypermobile.

Shin Splints

Shin splints are characterized by pain in the front of the shin bone. They are associated with exercise, usually running. Most people agree that the tibialis anterior muscle, on the front of the lower leg, is overrecruited which leads to this problem. This muscle, you may recall, is an ankle dorsiflexor: it points the toes or foot up when the leg is swinging through during gait.

In my experience, the reason this muscle is overworked is due to excessive effort to dorsiflex the ankle. This effort is caused by at least one of the problems we've been discussing: tight calf and soleus that it must work against; twisted femurs with feet that are pointing in the wrong direction, which necessitates increased effort by the dorsiflexors to lift the foot; or excessive heel strike, which means the dorsiflexors are turned on longer than if the foot were allowed to strike more through the midfoot.

Another possibility takes into account old ankle sprains that weren't correctly rehabbed. In this case, the ankle joint doesn't dorsiflex adequately, which prompts the tibialis anterior to work harder to move the joint.

As I've mentioned with the other foot problems, find and prioritize your specific issues.

Ankle Sprains

Ankle sprains are common, especially in sports. But some people's ankles sprain quite often. And some people's ankles continue to be painful long after the tissues should have healed. The most common sprain occurs when the ankle rolls to the outside. This is called an **inversion sprain**. The ligaments holding the ankle bones together become overly stretched or torn.

When the foot rolls to the outside, the talus (that irregularly shaped foot bone) pushes against the fibula. The fibula is then pushed to the outside as well separating it from the tibia, potentially stretching those ankle ligaments.

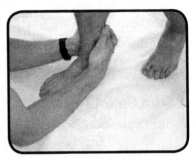

Squeezing the Ankle Joint
Figure 2.33 Squeezing the ankle joint together approximates the fibula and tibia, potentially reducing chronic ankle sprain pain.

If you have chronic painful ankle sprains, try gently squeezing your fibula and tibia together. In many cases this almost instantly eliminates pain (Figure 2.33).

I've found that many people's chronic sprains and ankle pain don't heal because these two bones aren't brought back together enough, which leaves the ankle joint looser and vulnerable to strains of the ankle ligaments.

If you've squeezed your ankle bones together and found it reduces your pain or you feel more stability, then you may want to tape these bones together. Squeeze the bones together while wrapping a snug piece of tape around them. This will help hold them together and is quite effective in most cases—especially prior to playing sports (Figure 2.34). Remember to consult your physician prior to taping your ankle.

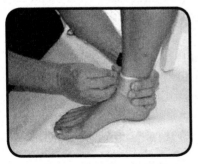

Chronic Ankle Sprain Taping
Figure 2.34 Taping the fibula and tibia together can reduce pain from chronic ankle sprains.

Another reason I prefer this taping technique is that it allows the foot and ankle to "learn" what they need to do to work properly. If we tape the entire foot and ankle complex (amounting to almost a cast), as you see in many athletes, it robs the body and especially the brain of learning to connect the foot to the knees, hips, and back. The term for this is **proprioception**. The key to taping an ankle, or any other part of the body, is to help stabilize it enough to function but not so much that the tape restricts it from moving. If you remember, many of the plantarflexor muscles of the lower leg act as guy wires to control the foot and ankle. That includes preventing the ankle from rolling out. So if you have chronic ankle sprain issues, then it makes sense that you would want your ankle and foot to be supported with more muscles earlier and longer throughout the gait cycle. The walking technique I've described above does just that.

If you have an acute sprain, then you do not want to wrap the entire ankle because fluid needs to escape. Instead, you need to tape the end of the fibula closer to the ankle joint using a piece of tape whose ends don't join together (Figure 2.35). This allows the ankle to function while removing stress from the injured ligaments. When stress is removed from tissue, it heals faster. But please make sure you consult your physician prior to taping. They are aware of all the factors contributing to your sprain and this technique may be counterproductive to those ends. Especially when inflammation is involved, consult your physician before attempting this taping technique.

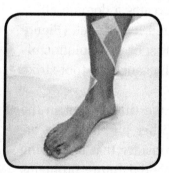

Acute Ankle Sprain Taping
Figure 2.35 Taping the fibula and tibia together can reduce pain from acute ankle sprains. Especially if swelling is present, it is important to keep the ends of the tape open so inflammation can leave the area.

Okay, we've gone over most foot and ankle problems. As with other parts of the body, functional problems express themselves as different injuries based on which tissues or joints are most susceptible. It's difficult to predict how they will manifest in each person, but it comes back to these same five basic principles in most cases.

Hopefully I've made a good argument that how you walk or stand; the unconscious contraction of your hip, calf, and foot muscles; and the shape of your feet and femurs all come together to create excessive stress

> **Proprioception** is your brain's ability to know how your body is positioned at any moment.

in the lower leg and foot. Each one of these issues alone can create problems, but one on top of another breaks down the foot and ankle system and creates chronic pain. That's why you need to understand the systemic problems feeding your particular pain. Solutions must involve more than one approach for most people with chronic pain.

Foot Orthoses

Orthotics is the branch of medicine that deals with creating foot inserts or orthoses. A foot orthosis (plural: orthoses) is the actual shoe insert. Many people just refer to orthoses as orthotics.

Foot orthoses are basically supports you can put in your shoe to help correct foot alignment issues. If done well, they are often quite effective in eliminating pain from foot, ankle, knee, hip, and even back issues. This is because the foot creates a domino effect of changes that can play out at the pelvis and lower back (Figure 2.36). Unfortunately, orthoses are often the first or only solution offered for problems that could be helped with changes in foot-strike patterns or other problem areas.

Granted, some people don't want to take the time or put in the effort to fix their mechanics and would rather just have the orthoses do the work. I get it. But please consider that taking the time to fix your issues will also avoid potential future problems in other parts of your body related to poor body awareness or mechanics. Trying to fix the root causes of foot, knee, hip, or back pain without using orthoses, can permanently correct chronic pain, and you will function better and prevent injuries down the road. Typically, this means correcting how we walk, among other things. I've found this approach to be very effective in resolving pain from plantar fasciitis, heel spurs, and other foot maladies. It is also part of my treatment for knee, hip, and back pain.

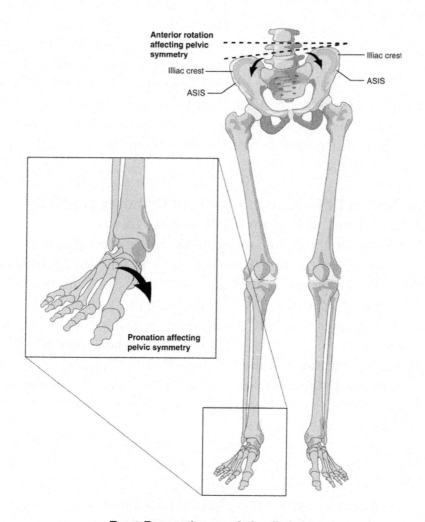

Foot Pronation and the Pelvis
Figure 2.36 Differences in foot pronation can affect pelvic alignment.

I want to emphasize that some people absolutely need the sup-

I recommend reading Gina Kolata's interesting article on the New York Times website (www.nytimes.com) "Close Look at Orthotics Raises a Welter of Doubts" which shows that no one really knows if or how orthoses help people.

port offered by orthoses. Usually, these people have very mobile feet or other problems they are unable to correct without them. If you are one of these people, the following information will hopefully help you understand how to assess your orthoses. Before reading further, I want to emphasize that I am not an authority on foot biomechanics and the effect of orthoses in fixing foot or ankle problems. There is a lot we don't know about orthoses (see text box) and so the information I'm presenting is based purely on my clinical experience.

Is There a Difference in How Foot Orthoses are Made?

Most orthoses are made (casted) with the foot in a non-weight-bearing position. Others are made by stepping on a platform to digitally assess the feet. However, these techniques are usually based on a principle that the foot should be casted in the "subtalar neutral" position. The central theme of this concept is that there is an ideal "neutral" position of the subtalar joint formed by the talus bone (on top) and the calcaneus bone (below). This theoretical position is called subtalar neutral. There are a couple problems with this approach, though. First, there isn't agreement about how best to measure where subtalar neutral is.[5] I can't even find the term on Wikipedia!

But even if a practitioner could somehow find subtalar neutral and keep the foot there during the casting process, then that means the orthoses are beginning to control the foot at subtalar neutral. To me, any motion beyond this ideal then potentially causes damage to the foot. And I think many orthoses casted in this position allow this to happen.

The casting system I use is Sole Supports. I like their approach because the foot is casted with a much higher arch (prior to subtalar neutral—whatever that is), which allows the foot to move into this theoretical subtalar neutral and then back out again. These orthoses are also adjusted to your specific weight. This makes sense to me, especially for those with hypermobile ankles and feet because these people need more control than most to keep them out of trouble. I am not being paid by Sole Supports to write this. It's just based on my experience and the fact that everyone I've casted for these orthoses are very happy they have them.

Something else you should know is that many companies use a prefabricated mold that most closely fits the needs of a patient's foot based on a pressure plate analysis or light model (whose program's premises may assume a subtalar neutral preference). Technically these are customized orthoses, not to be confused with *custom-made orthoses*.

Customized orthoses are prefabricated arch supports that are the closest match to the foot analysis. They may or may not be an adequate fit. They are often advertised as custom orthotics.

Custom-made shoe inserts fit one foot and one foot only—yours. Often there are differences between the left and right foot (mentioned earlier) that customized orthoses cannot adequately correct. Often the people selling the orthoses do not understand the differences between these terms, nor do they understand the premises behind the system they are selling. So you have to do your homework to find out which category your orthoses truly fit into and the reasoning behind how your orthoses are casted.

Why do I go into this detail? Because selling orthoses is big business. They are expensive, and you want to have as much information as you can prior to making your decision. I see lots of people every year who have paid too much money for their orthoses, only to find they do not adequately support their feet.

I do not automatically give people orthoses, even if they ask for them. This is because many foot, knee, hip, and back issues can be corrected without them. If we can't correct the issues, then I will fit them for a pair.

Tips for Assessing Your Foot Orthoses

So how do you know whether a pair of orthoses fits well? Assuming you need orthoses because you are unable to control the foot or ankle, I believe your orthoses should then provide complete support during the entire stance phase of gait. Here are three simple intuitive tests to find out if yours are doing the job.

Finger Test

Many orthoses are too soft and break down rapidly. A simple test can demonstrate this. Knowing that your body exerts at least its body weight with each step (and up to 3 times your weight), see if you can depress the arch of your orthoses your finger (Figure 2.37a & b). If your orthoses bend under this minimal force, just think what they're doing (or not doing) when you're walking or working! Remember the idea of subtalar neutral? If your orthoses collapse easily, then your feet are probably spending too much time beyond it. The thickness of your orthoses should be adjusted to your individual weight so they will always support your foot with the correct amount of flex.

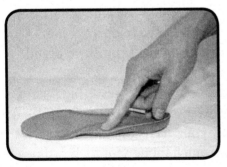

Finger Test
Figure 2.37a This orthosis collapses easily under minimal force.

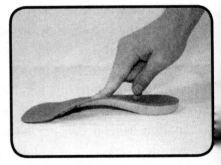

Finger Test
Figure 2.37b This orthosis withstands the minimal force produced by this test.

Standing Test

Here's another test. Stand in your orthoses and see if there is any gap between the shoe insert and your feet (Figure 2.38a & b). There should be no gap. If there is, then the orthoses are not supporting your feet when standing or during the midstance phase of gait.

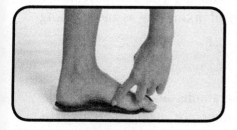

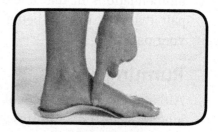

Standing Test
Figure 2.38a This image shows a gap between the orthosis and the foot.

Standing Test
Figure 2.38b This image shows the orthosis supports the foot when standing.

Heel Lift Test

Sit down with your orthoses under your feet. Raise your heel, bringing the orthosis with you (Figure 2.39a & b) similar to what would happen at the end of your gait cycle during heel off. Is there a gap between your orthosis and your foot? If so, then your shoe inserts may not be supporting your feet during the latter part of the walking cycle. This may be less of an issue because most of the weight is transferring to the balls of the feet at this point.

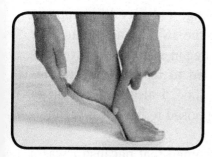

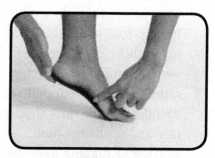

Heel Lift Test
Figure 2.39b Bringing the heel up with the orthosis shows support under the arch.

Heel Lift Test
Figure 2.39a Bringing the heel up with the orthosis shows a gap under the arch.

These are three simple tests you can perform on your current pair of orthoses, or if you're about to be fitted with a pair, then you can check out a typical sample and ask a few questions about how it is made and will fit your foot. My hope is that ultimately most of you will not need orthoses after you've read and tried the recommendations in this book. But if you do, you can purchase a pair that will have a better chance of fixing the issues causing your pain.

Running

Although I've run a couple of marathons and some half-marathons, I am not a professional runner nor even a serious one. Unlike so many elite runners, I am not gazelle-like. My personal goals for running are to take care of my joints and stay in shape so I can keep up with my kids as they grow older—not too lofty. I'll probably never run in the Boston marathon (unless I can keep my current speed when I'm 75!).

Prior to rethinking the foot and ankle, I ran using a heel-strike pattern in a pair of thick-soled shoes with orthoses. After every run my knees, hips, and back ached, sometimes for days. Luckily, I knew all the exercises to fix my aches and pains, but I couldn't figure out why the same problems came back again and again.

Soon after rethinking foot function, I decided I needed to test my theories on myself. My theory dictated that I needed a shoe that just protected the soles of my feet from debris of the road, perhaps offered the tiniest bit of cushioning, and very little support for my foot and ankle. I finally made the switch and pitched out my orthoses and running shoes and began running in my Converse® tennis shoes. After all, I needed to rely on my muscles rather than the external support of a shoe. I also didn't want to spend a fortune on a shoe that was supposed to have less technology and sophistication.

Initially, I made a huge mistake. I assumed that because I was a heel striker that I should start forefoot running. Well, after crippling pain in my calf muscles for weeks, I realized I simply didn't have the strength to make that change. After months of experimentation, I realized that some heel strike is okay, I just needed less than what I had been using. Now I run with a relaxed, rolling foot technique that employs a little heel and midfoot strike, then immediately rolls into a more solid midfoot strike. It's nearly a flat-foot strike.

If you try running in a minimalist pair of shoes, chances are if you just relax and let your feet find their way, they will. Don't overthink it; there is no one perfect way to run. There is only what is right for you. In minimalist shoes you will naturally avoid jarring heel strikes and other tendencies that don't feel right. Just start with low mileage, turn off the iPod, and become aware of what you are doing and what your body wants. You will find your way. You can eventually turn the music on again, but at first, just listen to your body.

Even with this modified technique, it took many months to build my plantarflexor strength to support this change. After all, I hadn't been using them for most of my life, and this technique requires their participation. Because of this lack of muscular development, I occasionally strained my calf muscles. One of the injuries occurred during my second 20-mile run when training for a marathon. After 14 miles of running, I stopped to refill my water, and my calves tightened up. I ran the last 6 miles with cramped calves and ended up straining/tearing one of my plantarflexor muscles. Not the most intelligent thing I've done. That put me out for almost 4 months, so I missed my marathon.

Two books that can help you change your running approach are **Chi Running: A Revolutionary Approach to Effortless, Injury-Free Running** by Danny Dreyer, and **The Barefoot Running Book: A Practical Guide to the Art and Science of Barefoot and Minimalist Shoe Running** by Jason Robillard.

The running technique I use has helped many clients too. Regardless of whether someone has foot, hip, knee, or back pain, I test their hips and feet to see how they walk. Most walk with an excessive heel strike and little to no gluteal contraction. First we work on their walking-gait pattern using the relaxed foot strike and activating the gluteals. Once walking is mastered, we then move on to running.

I begin my runners by jogging around the block. We run one block, working on integrating the principles they learned from their walking mechanics. Then we walk a block to reinforce again the mechanics we are trying to create. We continue alternating one block running with another block walking until they feel the connection between their gait, glutes, and foot-strike pattern. I ask them to build up slowly after that and to not think about speed at this time. Speed will come after you've learned to relax and run without breaking your body down.

Another idea I like to keep in mind is that the longer the contact stress with the ground, the more chance of injury. A strong heel-strike pattern seems to increase the force and contact time with the ground whereas a midfoot or forefoot strike seems to decrease both of these elements. This helps maintain a lightness in the foot strike that I believe decreases stress to the foot and ankle.

Barefoot Running

My personal preference is to have a pad between my feet and the road; however, many people prefer to run without even that. This is the current trend of barefoot running. Understandably, the scientific verdict is out regarding the safety of this philosophy.

At least one study shows that ground-reaction forces are typically lower in barefoot running as compared to wearing shoes.[6] This seems to be corroborated by my personal and clinical experience as I introduce patients to the concept of less shoe beneath their feet. The argument against barefoot running (or minimalist shoes) is that it introduces a potential for tendon or muscle strains. I can attest to that! After all, you are using more lower leg muscles to control your body. But I believe this vulnerability exists because these same muscles have been weakened through disuse due to the excessive heel-strike pattern. If you take your time to build your strength and endurance, you should be fine.

I want to emphasize that not everyone should change their shoe type or running style. Many people, including elite runners, do very well with thick-soled shoes and heel-strike running patterns. I'm merely introducing alternatives for those who have chronic injuries and are in need of answers to their pain. I'm reporting my clinical experiences, but there are many unknowns with this approach. Yes, barefoot running may be extreme to many people (including me), but I embrace the mechanics involved in this running style, that of less heel strike and earlier plantarflexor activation in the gait cycle. I still remember running in my first marathon (Grandma's Marathon in Duluth, Minnesota) and being passed by a man in bare feet. I thought, "That guy must be nuts!" as he sped off out of sight. Turns out he wasn't as nuts as I thought. Well, maybe just a little.

Putting It All Together

For many of you, your pain may completely go away with the techniques described in this chapter. You could continue with those exercises that eliminated your pain to keep it at bay, and that may be all the fix you need. I recommend you follow this course:

1. Discover which of the five mechanical issues are at work and rate how strongly they seem to manifest themselves in you. Choose the top two or three to focus on for the next week.

Poor walking habits _____
The shape of the thigh bones _____
The shape and mobility of the foot and ankle _____
Chronic calf and soleus contraction _____
Poor awareness or control of the foot muscles _____

2. If the mechanical exercises you've chosen to focus on aren't helping, then try the ones you haven't used.

3. Once your pain is reduced and your balance is restored, begin whittling the exercises down to a minimum to continue your pain-free status.

Fill out the following weekly log on the next page to help you track your issues, behaviors, and exercises and monitor your work. Under the "Behavior/Exercise" column, you will write down which goals you wish to work on. For instance, in the first column box (under Behavior/Exercise) you might write "Less heel strike while walking." In the "Desired Frequency" column you might write, "I will practice 5x/day for 2 minutes each time." In the "Actual Frequency" column, you will track how many times you actually practiced that behavior or exercise. Feel free to use the "Notes" section on this log to record tweaks you discovered that help you reduce your pain or perform the exercise better. Finally, in the "Pain" column, write down how each exercise has affected your pain. You many want to rate your pain on a 0 to 10 scale, 10 being intense pain and 0 being none. Track your pain immediately after the exercise and perhaps throughout the day. If you find your pain increases at a certain time of day (or after a particular behavior), then see if the exercise will reduce the pain. Tracking these patterns will help you clue in to what habits are irritating your feet.

If you have several exercises or behaviors to work on, then write them down in order of their ranking. That way, you address the most important one(s) first.

Behavior/Exercise Weekly Log

This is a log of the exercises and/or behaviors you will need to address during the week. Please fill the log in accurately.

Date: _____

BEHAVIOR/ EXERCISE	DESIRED FREQUENCY	ACTUAL FREQUENCY	PAIN	NOTES

1 C. Saltzman and D. Nawoczenski, "Complexities of Foot Architecture as a Base of Support," *Journal of Orthopaedic & Sports Physical Therapy* 21.6 (June 1995): 354–60.

2 Wegener, A. E. ,B. J. and R. M. "Effect of Children's Shoes on Gait: A Systematic Review and Meta-Analysis," *J Foot Ankle Res* 18.4 (Jan. 2011): 3.

3 Norman Doidge, *The Brain That Changes Itself: Stories of Personal Triumph from the Frontiers of Brain Science* (Penguin, 2007), 203–4.

4 W. D. and P. ,"Hallux Valgus and the First Metatarsal Arch Segment," *Physical Therapy* (Jan. 2010), 110–20.

5 Y. X. Chen, G. R. Yu, J. Mei, J. Q. Zhou, W. Wang "Assessment of Subtalar Joint Neutral Position: A Cadaveric Study," *Chin Med J* (Eng.) 121.8 (Apr. 20, 2008):735–39; A. M. Keenan and T. M. Bach, "Clinicians' Assessment of the Hindfoot: A Study of Reliability," *Foot Ankle Int.* 27.6 (Jun. 2006):451–60; T. J. Pearce and R. E. Buckley, "Subtalar Joint Movement: Clinical and Computed Tomography Scan Correlation," *Foot Ankle Int.* 29.7 (Jul. 1999): 428–32; K. Smith-Oricchio and B. Harris, "Interrater Reliability of Subtalar Neutral, Calcaneal Inversion and Eversion," *JOSPT* 12.11 (Jul. 1990): 10–15.

6 D. E. Lieberman, M. Venkadesan, W. A. Werbel, et al., "Foot-strike Patterns and Collision Forces in Habitually Barefoot versus Shod Runners," *Nature* 463.28 (2010): 531–35.

3 Corrective Exercises

I've been a few places like that where I've thought, "A **breakthrough** *is possible here. This is the place for the* **exercises** *that will bring me to* **where I want to be.**"

—**Joseph Campbell**

Most of the exercises you'll need to use are found in Chapter 2: Understanding Your Anatomy. The three exercises below are targeting important hip muscles which affect knee and consequently foot function. Although they are a bit removed from directly affecting foot and ankle performance, I think it's important to improve any function that involves the leg system. Gluteal function is definitely important to this system.

The following exercises are meant to develop strength and improve quality of motion. If you find a particular exercise difficult, decide whether this is due to range of motion or strength issues, or because the exercise is awkward to perform. Chances are it is due to weakness or movement dysfunction. Take that as a cue that you need help in that area and therefore should practice it until you've mastered it. Good form is critical.

If you find an exercise that feels good, then do it as often as you can. Trust your body, it knows what it likes! Add one exercise at a time to focus on getting it right and to test whether your pain is made worse by a particular exercise. If it is made worse, then either your technique is incorrect or it's not the right exercise for you. Pay attention to how you are performing the exercise. Read the instructions carefully and watch the video clips on the Fixing You website at www.FixingYou.net. Type in the code at the back of the book on page 100 to access the free clips. Once you are successfully performing the exercise, then layer on the next. Each time you add a new strengthening exercise, don't change anything else about your program. This way, you'll be able to isolate which exercise may be causing pain.

Just a little bit of strengthening is needed to effect a positive change. As always, *quality is more important than quantity.* Strengthening exercises only need to be performed one to three times per day.

GLUTEAL PUMPS

Purpose: This exercise restores strength to the gluteus maximus. This muscle often becomes weak, especially in the presence of tight muscles in the front of the pelvis. The hardest part of this exercise is to keep your spine from sagging down while exercising. Only work within a range that you can prevent this from happening.

The Fixing You Method: Assume a position on your elbows and knees with your spine flat and in a neutral position. Hold your spine in place by drawing your belly button in toward your spine. Squeeze your gluteals to raise one leg up in the air with your knee bent at 90 degrees. Try not to push your leg up with your foot or pull your leg up with your hamstrings (the muscles in the back of your leg). Pull it up by squeezing your gluteal muscles. Stop when you feel the maximal contraction of these muscles. Slowly lower your leg about ¼ to ½ inch. This ensures the glutes stay turned on and are doing the work. Maintain the gluteal contraction while you slowly pump your leg up and down. Make the gluteals fatigue. Perform 10–30 repetitions or until fatigue or failure (indicated if your hamstrings begin to fatigue instead of your gluteals). Switch sides.

Common problems:
• Don't arch your back to bring your leg up higher. Instead, stabilize your spine by drawing in your belly button.
• If your hamstrings cramp or fatigue, then you're using your hamstrings instead of your gluteals to lift your leg. Focus on pulling your leg up by squeezing your gluteus maximus (rear-end muscles). Keep your hamstrings relatively relaxed.

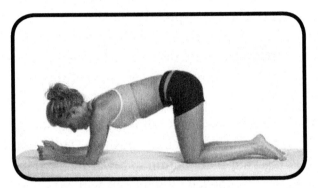

Glute Strengthening Begin

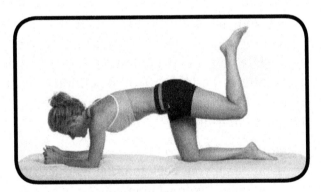

Glutet Strengthening Finish

STANDING HIP STRENGTHENING

Purpose: This exercise also strengthens the gluteal muscles and translates strength gains to walking or sports because performing it correctly requires stabilization of the entire body in a standing position.

The Fixing You Method: (If you have difficulty balancing, begin this exercise without an exercise tube and lightly hold on to a stable surface for assistance.) Stand and place an exercise tube or stretch band under both feet where your heels meet the arches of your feet. Raise the handles by bending your elbows as in the picture below. Raise your right foot off the floor approximately 1/2 inch. Slightly rotate your right knee outward while maintaining a square (neutral) pelvis and facing forward. Soften the left knee and be sure you are bearing weight through the arch or heel of the left foot, not the toes. While keeping your right foot lifted 1/2 inch from the floor, move it out to the side and then back in (4–12 inches). Make the movement smooth and slow while maintaining your square pelvis, soft left knee, and bearing your weight through the left arch or heel; maintain a tall spine without leaning. Perform 15 repetitions without allowing the right foot to touch the floor. Switch legs. Repeat 3 times on each leg.

Common problems:
• Back pain can result if your right leg is raised too far off the ground. Keep it elevated at 1/2 inch.
• Back pain can result if your pelvis is permitted to rotate while moving the raised leg. Maintain a neutral, forward-facing position.

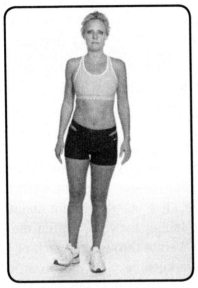

Standing Hip Strengthening
(no tube) Begin

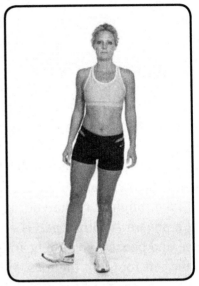

Standing Hip Strengthening
(no tube) Finish

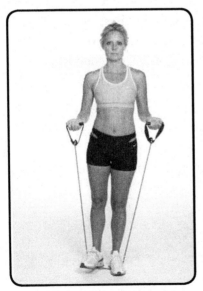

Standing Hip Strengthening
(with tube) Begin

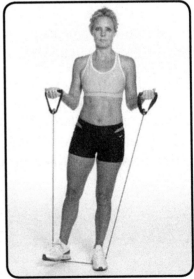

Standing Hip Strengthening
(with tube) Finish

LATERAL TUBE WALKING

Purpose: This exercise strengthens the gluteal muscles and translates strength gains to walking or sports because performing it correctly requires stabilization of the entire body while moving.

The Fixing You Method: (If you have difficulty balancing, begin this exercise without an exercise tube and lightly hold on to a stable surface for assistance.) Stand and place a circular exercise tube or stretch band around both ankles. Move to the side by walking the feet laterally keeping the knees soft and spine tall. The feet need only step slightly wider than your shoulders. Make the movement smooth and slow while maintaining your square pelvis and soft knees. Go about 10-15 feet in one direction and then return. Feel the hips working to stabilize and move your body. Repeat 2-3 times in each direction or until fatigue.

Common problems:
•   The trunk wobbles side-to-side while stepping. This diminishes the effort felt by the hips. Try to remain more rigid. To isolate the hips better, you can even put both hands on top of your head.
•   Bending the knees too much puts more effort on the thigh muscles than the hip muscles. Just a little softness in the knees is necessary.

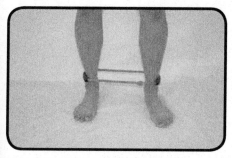
Lateral tube walking feet closer.

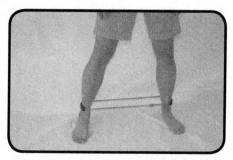
Lateral tube walking feet stepping wider.

FIXING YOU®: FOOT & ANKLE PAIN
GLOSSARY

anteversion-in terms of the thigh bone, anteversion refers to the internal rotation of the shaft of the thigh bone with respect to normal.

bunions-these form as a result of the long bone of the big toe moving outward often while the big toe moves inward.

calcaneus-the heel bone.

cuboid-one of the foot bones making up the arch.

cuneiform-a bone in the foot which helps form the arch. There are three cuneiforms.

dorsiflexion-the position of the foot when it is pointed upward toward the head.

eccentric contraction- the contraction of muscle while lengthening that muscle. For instance lowering yourself down to sit on a chair involves the eccentric contraction of the thigh muscles. They are lengthening while maintaining a contraction of the muscles.

external rotation-the outward rotation of an appendage.

fascia- connective tissue that binds muscles, nerves, and blood vessels together. It also blends with bone and is innervated.

femur-the thigh bone.

fibroblast- a type of cell that makes collagen which is a principal component of fascia.

fibula-one of the lower leg bones running from below the knee to make up the outer bone of the ankle.

gait cycle- term given to the overall walking strategy. The gait cycle is typically comprised of the heel strike, midstance, toe-off, and swing through stages.

gluteal-refers to the gluteus maximus and/or gluteus medius and/or gluteus minimus muscles.

hammertoes-when the middle joints of the toes migrate upward and more or less permanently remain there in a claw-like pattern.

heel spur-when a little bony lip develops where the the plantar fascia meets the heel bone.

homunculus-a representation of how our body is mapped out on our sensorimotor cortex.

hypermobile- excessively mobile or loose jointed.

internal rotation-the inward rotation of an appendage.

interosseous membrane-non-contractile tissue connecting the tibia and fibula bones.

inversion sprain-refers to injury of the ligaments holding the ankle bones together as a result of the foot rolling outwards.

ligaments-non-contractile tissue that connects bone to bone.

mechanoreceptor-a sensory nerve receptor that responds to changes in pressure and tension.

metatarsal-group of long bones connecting the arch to the base of the toes. These are usually numbered beginning with the big toe as the first metatarsal.

Morton's neuroma-a benign neuroma found on the nerve between the third and fourth toes typically.

myofibroblasts-a type of fibroblast combining structural features with the contractility of smooth muscle.

navicular-one of the bones of the arch.

patella-the knee cap.

plantar fascia-non-contractile tissue running from the heel bone to the bases of the toes.

plantar fasciitis-inflammation of the plantar fascia.

plantarflexion-the position of the foot when it is pointed down toward the floor.

pronation-term used when arch of the foot is flattened.

proprioception-refers to our ability to know where our body is in space. For instance, with eyes closed, knowing whether your arm is straight or bent.

reciprocal inhibition-a phenomenon where a muscle group on one side of a joint relaxes to allow the muscle group on the other side of the joint to contract.

retroversion-in terms of the thigh bone, retroversion refers to the external rotation of the shaft of the thigh bone with respect to normal.

sensorimotor cortex-the area of the brain that receives sensations from muscles and joints and relays the messages to the muscles to contract or relax.

supination-term used when the arch of the foot is elevated.

talus-one of the ankle bones that sits on top of the calcaneus and helps form the subtalar joint.

tibia-the lower leg bone that articulates with the femur to form the knee joint and the talus to form the ankle joint.

trigger points-a bundle of knotted muscular tissue which, when pressed, can cause pain locally or in a more distant area of the body.

voluntary motor cortex-the portion of the brain that controls our muscles.

About the Author

Following graduation in 1996 from the nationally ranked Krannert School of Physical Therapy at the University of Indianapolis, I practiced at a small sports and orthopedic clinic in Cortez, CO. Because the clinic had a small gym attached, I was able to progress patients to a higher functional level than if I were in a typical clinic. This unique model influenced me to consider personal training. I discovered that setting up therapeutic training programs for my patients helped them as much or more than any intervention I would perform manually.

I moved to Denver in 1999 and began working as a physical therapist and personal trainer at an exclusive health club in downtown Denver. While there, I continued to experiment with blending rehabilitation and personal training and added Pilates to my skill set. Within just a few months, I became the top-producing employee at the club. I held that position for the next four years until I opened my own studio/clinic.

In addition to providing individual client services, I also lead corporate seminars for injury prevention and correction. My focus on teaching employees the fundamentals of injury mechanics and practical ways to correct them has made me an effective force in changing corporate thinking about injuries, injury prevention, ergonomics, and fitness programs. I believe education is the key. I find that if you teach someone how the body works and why they experience pain, most people will be more diligent in helping themselves. No one wants to be in pain.

I am an active member of the American Physical Therapy Association, and I continue to explore combined rehabilitation and fitness techniques through professional development and continuing education. I live and work in Denver, Colorado with my wife and two young children.

References

Introduction opening quote:
Nechis, Barbara. 1993. Watercolor from the Heart. New York, NY: Watson-Guptill Publications.

Section 1 opening quote:
Yogananda, Paramahansa. 1997. Journey to Self-Realization. Los Angeles, CA: Self-Realization Fellowship.

Section 2 opening quote:
Chopra, Deepak. 1993. Creating Affluence: Wealth Conscsciousness in the Field of All Possibilities. San Rafael, CA: New World Library.

Section 3 opening quote:
Campbell, Joseph. 1991. The Joseph Campbell Companion: Reflections on the Art of Living. Ed. Diane K. Osbon. New York: HarperCollins.

Kendall, Florence, Elizabeth McCreary, and Patricia Provance. 1993. Muscles Testing and Function. Fourth edition. Baltimore, MD: Williams & Wilkins.

Sahrmann, Shirley A. 2002. Diagnosis and Treatment of Movement Impairment Syndromes. St. Louis, MO: Mosby.
Hanna, Thomas. 1988. Somatics: reawakening the mind's control of movement, flexibility, and health: Da Capo Press.

Myers, Thomas. 2009. Anatomy Trains: myofascial meridians for manual and movement therapists, 2nd edition: Elesvier.

To access your free video demonstrations of all exercises in this book, visit **www.FixingYou.net,** select the Foot & Ankle Pain book under "Books" tab at the top, and then click the "view Video Clips" button. Once on the video clip page, type in the code: **footstrike.**

Appendix A

The Schedule of Recent Experience*

This scale is designed to help identify and place a value on various events in your life that may cause stress.

Part A.

Please place an "x" next to the number of the event that you have experienced within the past year.

_____ 1. A lot more or a lot less trouble with the boss.

_____ 2. A major change in sleeping habits (sleeping a lot more or a lot less, or change in part of day when asleep).

_____ 3. A major change in eating habits (a lot more or a lot less food intake, or very different meal hours or surroundings).

_____ 4. A revision of personal habits (dress, manners, associations, etc.)

_____ 5. A major change in your usual type and/or amount of recreation.

_____ 6. A major change in your social activities (clubs, dancing, films, social visits, etc.)

_____ 7. A major change in church activities (a lot more or a lot less than usual).

_____ 8. A major change in number of family get-togethers (a lot more or a lot less than usual).

_____ 9. A major change in financial state (a lot worse off or a lot better off).

_____ 10. In-law troubles.

_____ 11. A major change in the number of arguments with spouse (a lot more or a lot less than usual regarding child-rearing, personal habits, etc.)

_____ 12. Sexual difficulties.

Part B.

On the space provided, indicate the number of times an event happened to you in the past two years.

_____ 13. Major personal injury or illness.

_____ 14. Death of a close family member (other than spouse).

_____ 15. Death of a spouse.

_____ 16. Death of a close friend.

_____ 17. Gaining a new family member (via birth, adoption, oldster moving in, etc.)

_____ 18. Major change in the health or behavior of a family member.

_____ 19. Change in residence.

_____ 20. Detention in jail or other institution.

_____ 21. Minor violation of the law.

_____ 22. Major business readjustment (merger, reorganization, bankruptcy, etc.)

_____ 23. Marriage.

_____ 24. Divorce.

_____ 25. Marital separation.

_____ 26. Outstanding personal achievement.

_____ 27. Son or daughter leaving home (marriage, off to college or university, etc.)

_____ 28. Retirement from work.

_____ 29. Major change in working hours or conditions.

_____ 30. Major change in responsibilities at work (promotion, demotion, transfer).

_____ 31. Dismissed from work.

_____ 32. Major change in living conditions (building a new house, remodeling, deterioration of home or neighborhood).

_____ 33. Marital partner beginning or ceasing work outside the home.

_____ 34. Taking on steep mortgage.

_____ 35. Taking on small mortgage.

_____ 36. Foreclosure on mortgage or a loan.

_____ 37. Vacation.

_____ 38. Changing school.

_____ 39. Changing line of work.

_____ 40. Beginning or ceasing formal schooling.

_____ 41. Marital reconciliation.

_____ 42. Pregnancy.

Instructions

For Part A, write down the values, listed below, for the events that happened to you in the past year (from your answers above).

For Part B, multiply the value, listed below, by the number of times the event happened to you (from your answers above), and write down your answer.

Then add your scores and write your total score below.

Part A

Life Event	Mean Value	Your Score
1.	23	_____
2.	16	_____
3.	15	_____
4.	24	_____
5.	19	_____
6.	18	_____
7.	19	_____
8.	15	_____
9.	38	_____
10.	29	_____
11.	35	_____
12.	39	_____

Part B

13.	53	_____
14.	63	_____
15.	100	_____
16.	37	_____

17.	39	_____
18.	44	_____
19.	20	_____
20.	63	_____
21.	11	_____
22.	39	_____
23.	50	_____
24.	73	_____
25.	65	_____
26.	28	_____
27.	29	_____
28.	45	_____
29.	20	_____
30.	29	_____
31.	47	_____
32.	25	_____
33.	26	_____
34.	31	_____
35.	17	_____
36.	30	_____
37.	13	_____
38.	20	_____
39.	36	_____
40.	26	_____
41.	45	_____
42.	40	_____

Your Total Score   _____

*The Schedule of Recent Experience (SRE) by Marion E. Amundson, Cheryl A. Hart and Thomas H. Holmes © 1981, "Reprinted by permission of the University of Washington Press".

Dr. Holmes and his colleagues found that the more change in your life, the more likely you are to become sick. According to his research, of the people with a score above 300 for the past year, 80 percent will become sick. A score of 150-299 means that about 50 percent of you will become sick. With a score below 150, about 30 percent of you will become sick.

Although this test wasn't designed to necessarily include musculoskeletal issues, I believe the rationale still applies. The more stress you have in your life, the more chronic tension is developed in your musculature. This tension often develops in patterns that contribute to chronic pain.

Some things to keep in mind are that the answers are subjective (what constitutes a "major change" to one person, may not be major at all to another). Also note that "good" events can deliver stress just as effectively as "bad" events. Regardless of what you think of the categories or point system used in this scale, I believe this test is valuable in helping identify potential stresses in our lives (good or bad) that may contribute to musculoskeletal tension which, in turn, can cause pain—stresses you may not have been aware of. I'm sure you can think of many other stresses not listed. It also gives us direction as to how much we should value that stress in terms of its potential effect in our lives.

If you scored high, it may be helpful to address those stresses in your life that seem to be driving up your score. Seeking help from a therapist to develop strategies to come to terms with your stress may be a good idea.

I believe the scale is also helpful because, after reading all the events, it heightens our awareness of potential events and/or stressors as they pop up in our lives. Ultimately I believe it is our *response to stress*, more than the stressor itself, that determines the effects of stress in our lives. Learning to anticipate and manage your responses to stress will have a dramatic effect on your pain.

CPSIA information can be obtained at www.ICGtesting.com
Printed in the USA
LVOW04s1828150915

454265LV00018B/986/P